DISASTER RESPONSE

MEDICAL AND HEALTH POLICIES

EDITED BY:
ARNAULD NICOGOSSIAN
AND BONNIE STABILE

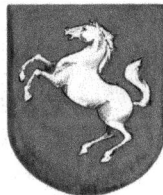

WESTPHALIA PRESS
An imprint of Policy Studies Organization

Also from Westphalia Press

westphaliapress.org

DISASTER RESPONSE

MEDICAL AND HEALTH POLICIES

DISASTER RESPONSE:
MEDICAL AND HEALTH POLICIES

Westphalia Press

Westphalia Press
An imprint of Policy Studies Organization
1527 New Hampshire Ave., NW
Washington, D.C. 20036
info@ipsonet.org

ISBN-13: 978-1-63391-163-5
ISBN-10: 1633911632

Daniel Gutierrez-Sandoval, Executive Director
PSO and Westphalia Press

Cover and Interior design by Taillefer Long at Illuminated Stories:
www.illuminatedstories.com

Updated material and comments on this edition
can be found at the Westphalia Press website:
www.westphaliapress.org

*Dedicated to the memory of our friend
and colleague David McCann*

IN MEMORIAM

DAVID G.C. MCCANN, MD, MPH, FAASFP, FAADM
(SEPTEMBER 29, 1960–AUGUST 7, 2011)

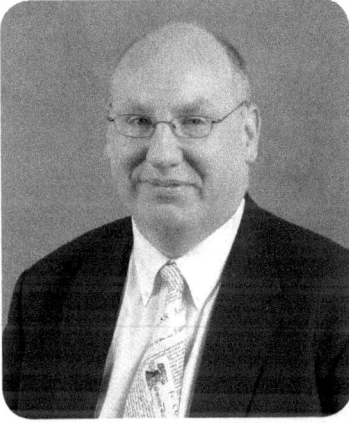

The Editors of the *World Medical and Health Policy* deeply felt the loss of a great professional, humanitarian, and one of our journal's strongest supporters and contributors. Dr. McCann was born in Boston, Massachusetts and died peacefully in Ontario, Canada, surrounded by his family after a short illness. Dr. McCann's main areas of research interest and practice were disaster medicine and public health, focusing on populations under extreme duress. David, a family practice physician from Dundas, Ontario, was an Associate Professor in the Department of Family Medicine at McMaster University, Ontario, Canada. He completed his Bachelor of Science at Dalhousie University, followed by postgraduate training at Memorial University of Newfoundland. He graduated in 2010 with a Masters of Public Health from the University of Massachusetts in Amherst. He practiced Family Medicine and Emergency Medicine in rural Southwest Georgia, where he was a Clinical Assistant Professor in the Departments of Family Medicine and Emergency Medicine at the Mercer University School of Medicine in Macon, Georgia, for almost 14 years. Dr. McCann was the Deputy Incident Manager for the Hamilton Health Sector in Ontario, Canada, where he also served as the Team Lead Physician at the Stonechurch Family Health Centre.

Since 2004 he served as the Chief Medical Officer of Florida One Disaster Medical Assistance Team with the U.S. Department of Health & Human Services and coordinated medical disaster preparedness and response in many world regions. He was involved in disaster response in Mississippi following Hurricane Katrina, and in Port-au-Prince, Haiti, after the 2010 earthquake. David also responded to the 9/11 tragedy in New York City: he boarded a train from Canada immediately after the event and was in New York City for the recovery phase of the tragedy. In 2011 he was installed as President of the American Board of Physician Specialists and was the Past Chair of the American Board of Disaster Medicine.

As a physician David was aware of his prognosis, but nevertheless continued to be productive, sharing precious time in the last days of life with his beloved family, colleagues, and the work that he loved. Throughout his ordeal David was sustained by his faith, passion for his profession and humanitarianism. He was in contact with his colleagues until the end, and provided wise counsel, encouragement, and focus for continued research and practice in the field of disaster medicine. The example of his life, work, and contributions will continue to offer guidance in the years to come in this new and rapidly evolving medical discipline.

David is survived by his spouse of 22 years Donna (neé Scott) and his beloved children Michael, Catherine, Maria, Danielle, and John-Paul; his brother Ronald McCann and sister Linda Johnston.

CONTENTS

INTRODUCTION

*"To have striven, to have made the effort, to have been true
to certain ideals—this alone is worth the struggle."*

Sir William Osler, MD

This book, a compilation of articles published in *World Medical and Health Policy* (WMHP), is dedicated to the celebration of the life of David McCann, a physician and humanitarian. August 8, 2014 marks the third anniversary of our loss of David McCann. He was a member of our Journal Editorial Advisory Board and a prolific author. Some of his publications are included in this book. Dr. McCann introduced WMHP to the many physicians dedicated to the practice of disaster medicine and humanitarian relief worldwide. He was instrumental in bringing together our *Center for the Study of International Medical Policies and Practices* (CSIMPP) in the School of Government, Policy and International Affairs at George Mason University with the *American Board of Physician Specialties* (ABPS), the official certifying body for the *American Association of Physician Specialists* (AAPS), to collaborate on educational activities in disaster medicine evidence-based practice and policies. Notably, Drs. Heidi P. Cordi, James W. Terbush, and Martin E. Thornton continue this collaboration through their participation in the WMHP Advisory Board. The Editors would like to also recognize the continued support and encouragement of William J. Carbone, Chief Executive Officer of the ABPS/AAPS, and his co-sponsorship of this publication.

Novel technologies such as global surveillance of disease threats, satellites, and computer modeling have resulted in a significant increase in survivability and decrease in damages from natural disasters. Yet preparedness remains a major factor in improving the readiness of communities and addressing disparities. The United Nations' (UN) has designated the second Wednesday of October annually as the *International Day for Natural Disaster Reduction*. This event is intended to remind professionals, communities, and governments to actively participate in addressing and reducing socioeconomic and medical suffering of victims. In 2014 the International Day for Disaster Reduction focuses its attention on an estimated one billion people living with some form of disability.

We hope that the knowledge and experiences described in this book will contribute in some modest way to the global effort in disaster reduction.

The Policy Studies Organization has played a significant role in nurturing WMHP, and we would like to thank them for their foresight in establishing the journal and their continued support as it grows.

Arnauld E. Nicogossian
Bonnie Stabile
Editors

I.
NATURAL AND HUMAN-MADE THREATS

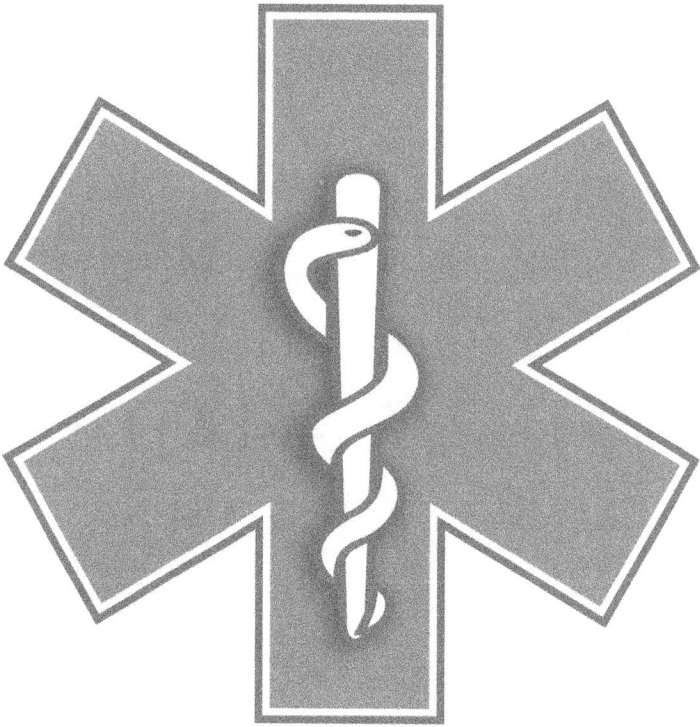

A REVIEW OF HURRICANE DISASTER PLANNING FOR THE ELDERLY

David GC McCann, *McMaster University School of Medicine*

INTRODUCTION

There is an old proverb that states, "He who fails to plan, plans to fail." Nowhere is the truth of this adage more evident than in the lack of disaster planning in some states along the U.S. Atlantic seaboard and Gulf Coast. These states' residents are at risk for hurricane landfalls annually between May 1 and November 30. In Florida, with its history of numerous hurricanes over the last century, local and state officials are highly motivated to maintain current, practical community disaster plans and to exercise them regularly. Unfortunately, the same cannot be said for some other states that have become complacent over the years as they were spared major hurricane landfalls. The tragic consequences of their complacency became abundantly clear in 2005 when Hurricanes Katrina and Rita ravaged the U.S. Gulf Coast. Too late did Louisiana and Mississippi realize the error of their ways to the detriment of their citizens.

The U.S. federal government, too, learned a bitter lesson from Katrina—disaster preparedness requires a major commitment of time and resources that cannot be relegated to "just in time" planning (Townsend et al. 2006). Comprehensive hurricane preparedness is essential to avoid catastrophic loss of life, particularly for the frail elderly (Silverman et al. 1995). The purpose of this paper is to discuss hurricane disaster planning with particular emphasis on challenges faced by the elderly who are among the most susceptible

3

to mortality and morbidity from tropical cyclones. In fact, 82% of Florida's elderly citizens live in exposed coastal areas and require special considerations both for evacuation and for sheltering in place (Silverman et al. 1995). This paper will focus primarily on disaster planning for elders with chronic diseases, those living in residential care, and those who are dialysis dependent.

WHAT IS A HURRICANE?

Hurricanes are tropical cyclones that arise in the Atlantic Ocean, the Caribbean Sea, and the Gulf of Mexico (Shatz, Wolcott, and Fairburn 2006). They begin as tropical depressions, which are organized systems of clouds and thunderstorms with a defined center of circulation and wind speeds of less than 39 mph. The developing storm draws energy from warm ocean waters, thus feeding the intensity of the winds and causing the storm to grow in size. At wind speeds of 39 mph up to 74 mph, the disturbances become tropical storms and are given names. Once wind speeds exceed 74 mph, a hurricane is said to exist. The Saffir–Simpson Scale is used by meteorologists to categorize hurricanes according to wind speed and potential for destruction (Table 1).

Hurricanes are one of nature's most destructive forces. Particularly for storms of Category 3 or higher, damage from wind can level homes, tear roofs off buildings, and turn flying debris into deadly projectiles. The torrential rains associated with hurricanes frequently cause widespread flooding, even hundreds of miles inland, especially in low-lying coastal regions. The most severe damage to the coastline, however, is caused by the storm surge that hurricanes engender. As the storm moves toward the coastline, it pushes massive amounts of ocean water ahead of it. The storm surge becomes ever bigger as the intensity of the storm increases and, especially if the hurricane makes landfall at high tide, can level the coastline for up to 10 miles inland (Alson et al. 1993).

Class	Winds (mph)	Tidal Surge (ft)
Category 1	74–95	4-5
Category 2	96-110	6-8
Category 3	111-130	9-12
Category 4	131-155	13-18
Category 5	>155	>18

Table 1. The Saffir–Simpson Hurricane Scale

Source: Alson et al. (1993).

THE ELDERLY AND DISASTER VULNERABILITY

In the wake of Hurricanes Katrina and Rita, it became clear that the elderly are disproportionately vulnerable to hurricanes. In fact, of the 1,330 people known to have died along the Gulf Coast, 71% of those in Louisiana were older than 60 years, 47% were over 75 years, and at least 68 persons died in nursing homes. Unfortunately, community disaster planning frequently fails to allow for the needs of older citizens before, during, and after hurricanes. In December 2005, the American Association of Retired Persons (AARP) convened a conference of governmental, scientific, and public sector experts to discuss ways to improve disaster preparedness for the elderly. The report which was issued after the conference noted several factors that predispose the elderly to morbidity and mortality from hurricanes (Gibson 2006). They include:

- The elderly frequently suffer from multiple comorbidities.

- They have functional limitations, including sensory, physical, and cognitive impairments.

    > According to the National Health Interview Survey (Schoenborn et al. 2006), visual impairment affects 13.9% of adults aged 65–74, 19.1% of those aged 74–84, and 30.3% of those aged 85 and over. Similarly, hearing loss affects 31.4% of adults aged 65–74, 43.9% of those aged 74–84, and 58% of those aged 85 and over.

    > Elderly people often suffer from loss of taste, smell, and/or

touch sensation, which leaves them more at risk for nutritional deficiencies and danger from fire or gas leaks (Murphy et al. 2002).

> Aging tends to diminish the efficiency of both sensory and muscular systems, rendering the elderly more at risk in disasters because of prolonged reaction time (Huxhold et al. 2006).

- They often take multiple medications.

    > Medications can increase risk for hypotension, falling, and confusion.

    > Sudden cessation of medication (e.g., running out of medications after a disaster and no physicians' offices or pharmacies are open to refill) can lead to life-threatening consequences.

- They usually rely on caregivers for assistance.

    > Many suffer from generalized "frailty," which can best be understood as a lack of biological reserve and resilience.

- Older citizens are much more susceptible to extremes of heat and cold that often accompany disasters (e.g., extreme heat in the hurricane season in Florida) (Oriol 1999).

- Many suffer from social isolation, especially those living alone and in rural areas.

    > After disasters, there can be significant worsening of elderly health issues as a result of the compounding loss of loved ones and friends, loss of income, loss of shelter (e.g., destroyed homes), loss of social status, etc. (Oriol 1999).

    > As a general rule, elderly people are much less likely to seek mental health counseling because they perceive mental illness as "weakness" (Oriol 1999).

In addition to the above challenges, Kilijanek and Drabek (1979) noted that the elderly do not seek financial support after disasters for a variety of reasons:

- They feel others may need the help more than they do.

- They do not like "welfare" handouts.

- They tend to seek insurance payouts and reconstruction of damaged property later than other adults, leaving their homes at risk from subsequent storms.

For disaster planning purposes, it is important to realize that the elderly are far from a homogeneous group. Gillick (1994) defined four groups of elders whose characteristics and differing needs must be borne in mind when planning for hurricanes:

1. *Robust elders*—those elders who maintain vigor in their later years. Although they may have health challenges, this group is able to fend for themselves as they do not suffer from functional disabilities.

2. *Frail elders*—those elders who have serious health problems and who use all of their capacity for survival. They have little or no functional capacity with which to respond to a disaster. Fernandez et al. (2002) give the following definition of frail elderly from an emergency management viewpoint:

Individuals aged 65 years or older with physical, cognitive, social, psychological, and/or economic challenges that will likely limit their ability to perform, or have performed for them, one or more of Activities of Daily Living or Instrumental Activities of Daily Living during and after a disaster.

Frailty is really a syndrome separate from the normal aging process—including unintentional weight loss, muscle weakness, slowed gait, exhaustion, and low physical activity (Gibson 2006).

1. *Elders with dementia*—loss of cognitive function renders these elders unable to understand what is happening during a disaster. They are not capable of making informed decisions and lack the ability to prepare for or respond to hurricanes.

2. *Dying elders*—for these elders, disasters can lead to serious questions of patient autonomy and control while increasing the burden on already stressed family members.

Keeping the unique challenges of elders in mind and recognizing that they are not a homogeneous group make disaster planning for older citizens very difficult. Nonetheless, using careful forethought and following basic principles of preparation and mitigation, there is no reason why hurricanes like Katrina should disproportionately affect the elderly in future. The public outcry after Katrina demonstrated that the U.S. electorate will not tolerate a lack of disaster planning from its elected officials in the future (Townsend et al. 2006).

An Overview of Disaster Planning Principles

Before discussing specific disaster planning priorities for the elderly, it is important to understand some general principles because a poorly planned response to a disaster is often a major problem in itself. This was amply demonstrated in the aftermath of Hurricane Katrina. Some of the early, seminal work in the area of disaster planning was undertaken at the Disaster Research Center (DRC) of Ohio State University in the 1960s. Quarantelli's group at DRC has contributed a great deal to the literature in this area and they define disaster planning as "...an attempt, prior to the actual occurrence of a crisis, to facilitate recognition of emergency demands and to make more effective the community response" (Dynes, Quarantelli, and Kreps 1981). They enumerated some important characteristics of disaster planning which should be kept in mind (Dynes, Quarantelli, and Kreps 1981):

1. **Disaster planning is a continuous process**: an unrevised, out-of-date plan is worse than no plan at all because it engenders a false sense of preparedness—the so-called "paper plan syndrome." In fact, well-prepared communities make it a policy to develop a disaster plan, exercise it until it breaks, redesign the plan to fix the inherent flaws, and then exercise it again (until it breaks). The importance of this iterative approach to disaster planning cannot be overstated.

2. **Planning seeks to reduce the unknowns in problem situations:** one tries to anticipate problems that will crop up and provide solutions in advance that will mitigate the potential effects. Hurricanes cannot

be stopped but the damage to infrastructure and potential loss of life can be mitigated through careful planning.

3. **Planning tries to foster appropriate, effective actions in a crisis:** it may seem natural to rush right out after a hurricane and start "doing something" but it is far more effective and efficient to first gather necessary information. This so-called "rapid needs assessment" allows the disaster response to be tailored to actual needs on the ground in the disaster zone and avoids well-meaning but ill-advised impulsivity.

4. **Planning should be based upon what is most likely to occur:** designing a disaster plan based upon idealistic, naive thinking is distinctly counterproductive. One must recognize and plan for what people are likely to do and not create elaborate plans that try to get the population to do things that do not "come naturally" when under duress.

5. **Planning must be grounded in fact, not supposition and myth**: there are numerous false assumptions about disasters that have been debunked in the literature but that are still prevalent in the minds of planning officials, such as (Auf der Heide 2000):

    - people will panic (this is actually rare)—in fact, with hurricanes people often refuse to evacuate despite mandatory evacuation orders (including the elderly);

    - people will be immobilized by fear ("disaster stunned")—actually, the local community usually pulls together immediately and helps one another;

    - local organizations will be paralyzed—local groups become the focus for community response in the aftermath of hurricanes;

    - antisocial behavior will be common (looting, etc.)—this actually occurs in a minority of situations (New Orleans after Katrina notwithstanding);

    - community morale will be low—often hurricanes cause dramatic "community mindedness" and laudably altruistic responses from local citizens.

6. **Planning should focus on broad principles, not on minute details**: the so-called "all hazards" approach to disaster preparedness. Rather than develop detailed, specific plans for each possible disaster, instead basic principles of action should be the focus of attention. In fact, detailed tome-like disaster plans are often developed for Joint Commission accreditation but are uniformly ignored in practice because no one has read them and they are not practical to implement.

7. **Planning is an educational activity**: part of the purpose of planning is to engage stakeholders in a process that heightens awareness and fosters resilience in the face of a crisis. Such an educational approach to disaster planning empowers stakeholders with the "can do" attitude which is so important in crisis management.

8. **Planning always faces resistance**: especially when no calamity has occurred for many years, it is notoriously difficult to engage communities in expensive, time-consuming disaster planning and exercising.

The aforementioned general principles for disaster planning will be important when designing hurricane disaster plans for elderly citizens, especially those with chronic illnesses, those residing in residential care, and those who are dialysis dependent.

The Incident Management System

Those who have a fiduciary responsibility to care for the elderly should have an effective system by which to manage disasters effectively. Clear lines of authority among federal, state, and local governments are critical to effective disaster response. The best method to ensure proper communication and chain of command in any disaster situation involves the Incident Management System (IMS) (McCann 2009a; 2009b). The IMS was originally developed by firefighters responding to wildfires in Southern California back in the 1970s. They discovered that fighting fires over a widespread area required a system of command and control to allow proper coordination and safety of responders. To properly coordinate operations at a disaster site, it is critical that all responders follow a clear chain of command. The IMS provides just such military-style command and control (see Figure 1). Unfortunately, many groups who care for the elderly are unaware of the IMS and how to operate within its structure (especially nursing homes and other residential care facilities). Unless the IMS structure is rigorously followed during a hurricane response, people get lost, hazards get missed, and chaos reigns. Therefore, the IMS is absolutely essential for effective disaster planning for the elderly.

Whoever arrives first at a disaster scene becomes the de facto Incident Commander (IC) until someone more senior arrives. He is assisted by Chiefs of the four Sections under him: Operations, Planning, Logistics, and Finance/Administration.

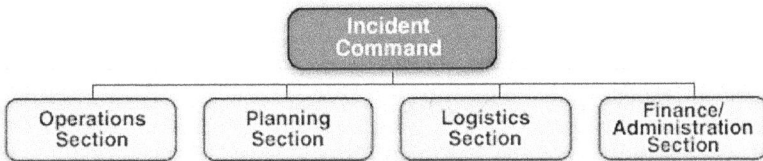

Figure 1. The Incident Management System Basic Structure
Source: Federal Emergency Management Agency (FEMA) Emergency Management Institute IS-100.

The roles of each of these players are:

Incident Commander (IC): the person who decides the objectives at the disaster scene, determines strategies to fulfill objectives, sets priorities, and has overall responsibility for the disaster (**The Boss**).

Operations Chief: leads the Operations Section, which is responsible for conducting the operations to achieve the objectives as determined by the IC, and decides on tactics and controls use of resources (**The Doers**).

Planning Chief: leads the Planning Section and whose task it is to develop the daily Incident Action Plan in consultation with the IC. This plan determines the activities for that day, tracks resources, collects data, and maintains appropriate documentation (**The Planners**).

Logistics Chief: leads the Logistics Section, which is responsible for providing the resources and services needed by the Operations Section (**The Getters**).

Finance/Administration Chief: leads the Finance/Administration Section, which is charged with monitoring costs and doing cost analysis, accounting, procurement and contracts, and pays the responders (**The Payers**).

Two key characteristics of the IMS are that it is scalable and flexible. So, in a small incident (not a disaster), the IC may be the "whole team." In a larger incident, it is likely the IC would populate all four Section Chiefs noted above. Depending on the amount of work, the chiefs may need a significant number of people in each of their sections. Here is another key concept in the IMS—span of control. The span of control refers to the number of people who may report directly to one supervisor. The number varies between three and seven persons—ideally five. If one has more than seven people in his down line, another branch of the IMS under that person must be created so that the maximum span of control principle is not violated. Further, each person reports to one and only one supervisor—a concept known as unity of command (McCann 2009a; 2009b). The United States has developed the National Incident Management System (NIMS), which relies on the IMS for its structure. NIMS, in turn, is a critical part of the National Response Framework (NRF), which describes the federal mechanisms of response in disasters requiring federal assistance. Disaster medical personnel working within the United States must understand NIMS and the NRF in order to function effectively (McCann 2009a; 2009b). Similarly, those who are dedicated to the care of the elderly must be able to function within the NRF and NIMS in the event of a hurricane if they are to do the most good for their clients. Therefore, administrators of residential facilities for the elderly and groups that contribute to elder care (e.g., Alzheimer's Association, AARP, etc.) need to understand their roles within the NRF and NIMS in times of disaster.

In a mass disaster situation, the exigencies of the situation might require multiple ICs in various sites over a large area. In this case, a unified command (UC) is formed and the various ICs report to the UC. A complete discussion of a large IMS such as a unified command is beyond the scope of this paper. A final word on the IMS—there is a truism well known in disaster management circles—for every five minutes one delays instituting the IMS structure in a disaster, it will require an extra 30–60 minutes to get the situation under control later (McCann 2009a; 2009b). Given the often precarious health of frail elders, the more quickly the IMS is enacted, the greater the likelihood that elders will be spared significant morbidity and mortality.

How Disaster-Prepared Are the Elderly?

A fair question to ask would be—just how disaster-prepared are the elderly in general? A study carried out by Cherniack and coworkers sought to answer this important question (Cherniack et al. 2008). The authors surveyed 547 ambulatory elderly patients attending a Florida urban teaching hospital's geriatric clinic in the wake of the 2005 Hurricane Wilma. The 25-question survey tool asked the participants if they:

- followed the American Red Cross guidelines for hurricane preparation:

  > specifically queried about what supplies they had, whether they planned to evacuate, and whether they used storm-resistant window shutters,

- understood the meaning of hurricane watches and warnings,

- had fallen, missed medications, or missed doctor's appointments in the two weeks after Hurricane Wilma.

One hundred and five patients were asked about the same three health outcomes (falls, missed medications, and missed doctor's appointments) 1.5 years later. The results of the survey demonstrated:

- Two thirds of participants were missing at least one hurricane supply item (a multivariate analysis showed no relationship between participants' demographics and the acquisition of supply items).

- Thirty-six percent planned to evacuate, but of those, only 56% had a developed evacuation plan.

- Sixty-three percent had storm-resistant shutters, but only 46% of those could install them.

- Twenty-eight percent had gas-powered generators, but only 46% of those knew how to operate a generator (a potentially life-threatening situation given explosion risk, carbon monoxide vapor, etc.).

- Interestingly, subjects after Hurricane Wilma missed significantly fewer doses of medication (3.4% missed after the hurricane versus 6.7% baseline, $p < 0.0001$), and fell significantly less often (8.8% after the hurricane versus 12.9% baseline, $p < 0.0001$).

- Subjects missed significantly more doctor's appointments after the hurricane (11.6% versus 0.1%, $p < 0.0001$).

Clearly, even Florida's ambulatory, hurricane-experienced seniors are not adequately disaster-prepared. Why should this be the case in a state so thoroughly familiar with hurricane devastation? There are a number of possible reasons:

- State and local officials in charge of hurricane planning have not adequately educated the elderly public or their educational efforts and methodologies have been ineffective.

- The elderly public is so "hurricane hardened" that they do not care enough to prepare.

- The public has developed a perception that "the government will take care of me" (entitlement).

- The public has developed a fatalistic sense that "when my number's up, it's up...."

- They have so many daily things to worry about (taking multiple medications, doctor's appointments, etc.) they neglect to plan for hurricanes.

In all probability, each of these possibilities plays a role in the woefully inadequate hurricane preparedness of the elderly. Nonetheless, it behooves hurricane disaster planners to reach out to the elderly in new and innovative ways to improve their hurricane awareness.

The Elderly with Chronic Diseases

Even robust elders usually have to deal with one or more chronic illnesses such as hypertension or diabetes. Unfortunately, post-hurricane treatment of chronic diseases in the elderly had not been a public health or medical priority for disaster planners until the experience of Hurricanes Katrina and Rita radically altered their viewpoint. Now it is clear that managing patients with chronic diseases after hurricanes must become a public health and medical priority. It is known that 80% of adults aged 65 and older have at least one chronic illness and 50% have at least two (Ford et al. 2006). In particular, almost 50% of elderly people have hypertension, 36% have arthritis, 20% have coronary artery disease, 20% have cancer, 15% have diabetes, and 9% have had a stroke (CDC 2004).

In the immediate aftermath of those two storms, the Centers for Disease Control and Prevention (CDC) carried out a limited needs assessment in evacuation shelters during September 10–12, 2005. They found that the majority of health needs in evacuees aside from injuries involved medication resupply, oral health problems, and chronic health conditions. Of the top 10 reasons for health visits in this evacuee population, the CDC found that four were related to chronic illnesses. Hypertension and cardiovascular diseases topped the list with an incidence of 108.2 per 1,000 residents. Next in frequency was diabetes at 65.3 per 1,000 residents. Farther down the list came preexisting psychiatric disorders (50/1,000) and asthma COPD (27.5/1,000) (CDC 2005).

15

Those suffering from chronic illnesses are at increased risk for exacerbations of their underlying diseases after hurricane disasters for a variety of reasons (Mokdad et al. 2005):

- lack of food leading to malnutrition,
- lack of clean water leading to dehydration,
- lack of electricity leading to temperature extremes (no air conditioning),
- physical and mental stress,
- injury,
- exposure to infections,
- lack of medical care,
- lack of medication and no way to obtain refills (pharmacies closed).

To properly plan for the post-disaster needs of chronically ill elders, Mokdad and colleagues (CDC 2005) noted that more information is needed by planners, specifically:

- pre-disaster rates of adverse health outcomes and the overall burden of chronic disease in hurricane-prone zones;
- awareness of the immediate needs of those with chronic illnesses;
- assessment of the basic and surge capacities of healthcare delivery systems to treat and manage those with chronic diseases in hurricane-prone areas;
- assessment of the ability to rebuild critical healthcare infrastructure after the disaster.

The same authors recommended the development of a surveillance tool that can determine the needs of the chronically ill before, during, and after a hurricane disaster. The surveillance tool would need:

- the ability to determine baseline size, functional status, and specific needs of vulnerable populations in hurricane-prone areas;
- the ability to assess on-the-ground needs and actual response during a disaster;
- the ability to monitor long-term effects after the disaster.

In 2004 (prior to Hurricane Katrina and disconcertingly prescient in their choice of study locale), the same group at the CDC (Ford et al. 2006) had trialed a surveillance system that already existed, the Behavioural Risk Factor Surveillance System (BRFSS) (Nelson et al. 2001), to determine the chronic disease burden in the greater New Orleans area. Looking at adults aged 18 and older, they found that 9% had diabetes, 4.6% had angina/coronary artery disease, 3% had had a myocardial infarction, 2% had had a stroke, and 6.3% had asthma. A quarter of all adults in the BRFSS had at least one of the aforementioned illnesses. The BRFSS satisfied some of the criteria for a chronic illness surveillance tool, but by no means all of them. The development of a more robust surveillance tool and a means to roll it out in hurricane-prone states are urgent research priorities.

So, how can disaster planners better prepare for the medical needs of elders with chronic illness in the aftermath of hurricanes? Aldrich and Benson at the CDC (Aldrich and Benson 2008) make a number of salient recommendations:

- Foster strong relationships among public health agencies, aging services organizations, emergency response personnel, and county and state Emergency Operations Centers (EOCs) in advance of disasters to ameliorate communication, coordination, and effective response (Gibson 2006) (during a hurricane disaster, such an "aging services network" would be able to reach out to the elderly with food, water, shelter, or medications).
- Have redundant communications systems and keep essential records in two different locations.
- Use Global Information System (GIS) mapping to mark areas with higher concentrations of the elderly.
- Have a specific emergency plan for the elderly and have shelters that cater to their needs.
- Have an evacuation system in place that includes transportation of their medications and other medical supplies, as well as a way to evacuate their pets (the elderly will frequently refuse to evacuate

if it entails leaving their pets behind).

- Provide better education on hurricane preparedness and evacuation planning in media that are easily accessible and understandable by the elderly, especially those with disabilities.
- Have a secure photo ID system in place that will allow healthcare personnel and senior service workers to gain access to their elderly patients in a disaster situation.
- Develop an emergency support system for in-home health services for the elderly.
- Develop an emergency respite care and communications plan for in-home caregivers of elderly patients.
- Develop a list of volunteers (with appropriate ID badging) for use in disasters.
- Partner with local restaurants to provide food to the elderly after hurricane.
- Improve identification and tracking for the elderly and for their medical records (the latter would be improved when the nation moves toward mandatory electronic medical records).

Implementing the above suggestions would offer significant improvements for disaster planning for the elderly with chronic diseases. Local and state officials, especially EOCs, need to make these recommendations a reality during the inter-disaster phase of their planning so that the response to a hurricane will be more efficient.

The Elderly in Residential Care Facilities

Disaster planning for the elderly living in residential care facilities such as nursing homes and assisted living facilities is particularly challenging. Negative experiences with Hurricanes Katrina and Rita in 2005 stimulated critical rethinking of this issue, resulting in a number of important recommendations for future planning (Polivka-West and Berman 2008):

- Nursing home disaster plans must be integrated into local, state, and federal disaster response plans (Dosa et al. 2008).

- Residential care facilities must be given the same priority status as hospitals for return of power and other essential services after a hurricane. For example, many Emergency Operations Centers (EOCs) (the hub of disaster response operations at the community, county, state, or regional level—also known as EOCs) do not recognize nursing homes as healthcare facilities—they consider them private entities "on their own" (Dosa et al. 2008).

- They must maintain effective communication between the facilities and the EOCs, relying if necessary on satellite phones and ham radio operators when land phone lines and cell phones are knocked out.

- Facilities should plan on hardening their physical plant structurally and plan for effective emergency power generation in the aftermath of the storm.

- Facility administrators should have knowledge of how the facility is situated with regard to storm surges, flood plains, and wind resistance. Despite a beautiful view, facilities overlooking the ocean are at far higher risk than those inland.

- The plan should include effective methods for communicating with residents' families and facility staff before, during, and in the aftermath of hurricanes.

- The facilities should test the facility disaster plan with regular drilling. In particular, test the plan with respect to the cognitively impaired and those with special needs such as dialysis.

- They need at least seven days worth of supplies, medications, and medical equipment on hand for residents and at least two weeks worth of food for everyone sheltering at the facility (residents, staff, and their families).

- They should plan for elderly people living in the community to be admitted in advance of the storm. Also plan for staff and their families to shelter in the facility. For example, a 500-bed nursing home in Miami ended up sheltering over a thousand in their facility, some of whom were elders abandoned by their families with no medical information or medication lists (Silverman et al. 1995).

- Patients need adequate identification (preferably wrist bands with bar codes), especially since many residents will be new and unfamiliar to the staff (Silverman et al. 1995).

- There needs to be a plan for having no elevator service and inadequate staff (Silverman et al. 1995).

- Plan for no power or air conditioning—elders have poor temperature homeostasis and become easily dehydrated in hot temperatures characteristic of the hurricane season. They will need significantly increased volumes of fluid and lots of ice (Silverman et al. 1995).

- Facilities will require at least five gallons of potable water per resident per day for drinking and two to three gallons of nonpotable water per toilet flush (Silverman et al. 1995).

- Facilities will require emergency power generators and fuel for at least a week of continuous generator operation (Silverman et al. 1995).

- Facilities should have year-round cross-training of all staff. This allows effective deployment of decreased numbers of staff to perform needed tasks normally not part of their job description (Laditka et al. 2009). Especially important after a hurricane are emotional support and ongoing physical care of the residents.

The biggest dilemma for administrators of residential care facilities facing a hurricane is whether or not to evacuate their residents. To quote a nursing home administrator, "The decision whether you evacuate or don't is the toughest decision and there is no government assistance, there are no guidelines" (Aldrich and Benson 2008). Evacuation of elderly residents is extremely difficult for a number of reasons:

- Elderly residents tend to have significantly more functional limitations than their community-living peers.

- Those evacuated demonstrate a 2–3-fold increase in falls over the next three months post-evacuation.

- Evacuated residents have altered sleeping and eating patterns.

- The elderly have increased dependency and insecurity.

- Modern nursing homes have increased acuity of patients compared with the past, making evacuation more logistically challenging.

- Evacuees suffer exacerbations of chronic disease and preexisting mental illness, including depression and psychosis (Castro et al. 2008).

- The decision of whether or not to evacuate residential care facilities must be based on a number of variables (Aldrich and Benson 2008):

- The severity of the approaching hurricane—one is much less likely to plan evacuation for a Category 1 hurricane, but one would be foolhardy not to consider leaving in the face of a Category 5 hurricane. Unfortunately, nature is inherently fickle. For example, Florida Gulf Coast residents went to bed in 1994 thinking Hurricane Opal was a Category 1 storm and awoke to a dangerous Category 4 monster, leaving no time for evacuation.

- The threat of storm surge, which is dependent on the strength of the storm at landfall and the facility's proximity to the coast as well as its height above sea level.

- The "hardness" of the physical plant—facilities built to hurricane standards will withstand high winds better than older facilities with less stringent building standards.

- Previous evacuation experience of the facility.

- Logistical issues such as availability of transportation (buses), a place to evacuate to, etc.

Evacuating elderly residents in advance of a hurricane requires tremendous effort and careful planning. It is a time-consuming and expensive proposition since it requires transport, not only of the residents but also of staff, medical equipment, disposable supplies, food and water, etc.

Therefore, the administrator of the facility must evaluate the risk to residents of evacuating versus sheltering in place (Aldrich and Benson 2008).

In another study, the authors compared 11 Louisiana nursing homes that sheltered in place during Hurricanes Katrina and Rita and 15 other nursing homes that chose to evacuate (Dosa et al. 2007). Of those who evacuated, 3/15 (20%) suffered no adverse consequences, 5/15 (33%) encountered transportation problems, 3/15 (20%) had staffing difficulties, 2/15 (13%) had issues in dealing with the shelters they evacuated to, and 6/15 (40%) suffered morbidity and mortality of their elderly residents. In contradistinction, for the 11 nursing homes that chose to "ride out the storm," 2/11 (18%) had no adverse consequences, 5/11 (45%) suffered facility damage from the storms, 4/11 (36%) had staffing difficulties, 8/11 (73%) noted supply difficulties (e.g., power, water, medications), but only 1/11 (9%) suffered morbidity and mortality among their residents. Clearly, those who evacuated suffered a disproportionate morbidity and mortality burden among their residents, while sheltering in place had significant issues with supplies (73%) but little or no morbidity/mortality among their elders. This data strongly suggests that sheltering in place is the safer option, provided the facility "stocks up" adequately and allows for emergency power generation during the inevitable power outages after the hurricane. One of the nursing home administrators included in the study made the following observation, "When you start moving [the residents] out, it's a tremendous burden, it's very hard. They're pulled and tugged. Their bodies are contorted into those buses. They're so heavy. It's not an easy thing to do that. And how much of a toll it takes on the residents just to do that to them" (Aldrich and Benson 2008). Another study by Castro et al. (2008) noted similar findings. Among those facilities that experienced a resident death, an average of 74.29 (SD = 31.77, n = 7) residents were evacuated. Among facilities that suffered no resident mortality, an average of 36.22 (SD = 40.68, n = 117) residents were evacuated—a statistically significant difference (p = 0.01). Similarly, a statistically significant difference was found when bus use for evacuating residents was examined. Those facilities that experienced a resident death averaged 85.71% bus use to evacuate residents (n = 6) versus 39.66% bus use (n = 46) for those facilities that did not suffer resident mortality (p = 0.04).

The following transportation issues were noted for evacuation (Dosa et al. 2007):

- Bus vendors failed to live up to their contracts to evacuate, especially local vendors within the hurricane evacuation zone.

- Buses often were not outfitted to handle wheelchairs and stretchers.

- Bus trips were often prolonged and hard on the frailest elders.

- Residents with cognitive impairment were difficult to load onto buses.

Suggestions to improve the transportation challenges include (Dosa et al. 2007):

- Contract with bus vendors outside of the likely evacuation zone, particularly those in the general area of the place to which the elders will be evacuated (local vendors often refused to provide service or had no bus drivers because they had evacuated themselves).

- Prior to the hurricane season, build ramps to allow wheelchair access to the buses.

- Evacuate the frailest residents in nursing home vans or send them to hospitals outside the likely evacuation zone well in advance of evacuating the rest of the facility.

- Have family members evacuate their own residents, especially those with cognitive impairment who are able to ambulate on their own.

Staffing issues were also noted for evacuation, including (Dosa et al. 2007):

- Staff refused to leave their family behind.

- Staff often failed to show up for work or flatly refused to evacuate.

- Staff had no financial incentive to stay at work.

- Nursing shortages were particularly acute.

The authors suggested the following to ameliorate staffing difficulties (Dosa et al. 2007):

- The facility should offer to shelter and evacuate their staff's immediate family members.

- The facility should facilitate organization of volunteers at the evacuation shelter destination in advance of the storm.

- The facility should offer financial incentives to staff to encourage work during the hurricane.

- The facility should arrange visiting nurses at the evacuation shelter in advance of evacuation.

Evacuating the facility is only half the battle. The place to which the residents will be evacuated also has potential issues that can cause problems, including (Dosa et al. 2007):

- Most nursing home residents require more acute care than hastily concocted shelters can provide. (For example, a high school gymnasium will not offer the kind of amenities required by a bed-ridden, frail, demented resident.)

- Potential shelters are often across state lines. Medicaid payments may not be made between states, making it likely that future evacuations to such facilities will be denied on a "lack of funding" basis.

The authors suggest the following potential solutions to the shelter issues (Dosa et al. 2007):

- A two-tiered method of evacuation—shelter locally for the first 48 hours, such as a local high school gymnasium. Such facilities would not be acceptable for prolonged sheltering but would allow a quick return to the residential facility in the event of minor damage or a "near miss" storm. Then, if unable to return to the facility in 48 hours, evacuate to an appropriate facility outside the evacuation zone capable of providing necessary care to the residents (e.g., another nursing home, a hospital, a military base, etc.).

- Payment issues should be resolved quickly so that the "door stays open" for future evacuations.

Just as there are issues with evacuation, there are issues with sheltering in place. Dosa et al. (2007) found the following facility issues:

- Generators (if there were any) often ran for only a few days and did not provide sufficient power for all needs (especially air conditioning).

- Nursing homes were usually not a priority for return of power and other essential services.

- Safety issues after the storm were a potential problem—people showing up in search of narcotics, etc.

- Supplies were used up much more quickly than anticipated, and there was no way to obtain a resupply for days/weeks after the storm.

They suggested the following ideas to mitigate the aforementioned issues (Dosa et al. 2007):

- Facilities should upgrade their generators so that they can run all electrical needs (especially air conditioning) for at least a week (NB—many facilities have their generators on the ground level—this is a poor design when water rises).

- Facility plans should be integrated into local and state disaster plans (as mentioned previously in this paper).

- Local police and National Guard should be part of the plan to provide security after the storm (National Guard is more likely to be useful as local police, if available, and will be otherwise occupied in multiple sites).

- Test the facility's emergency supply regularly since a seven-day supply may only last a couple of days with staff and resident families cosheltering with residents.

Finally, staffing issues were problematic for facilities that sheltered in place. In particular, it was noted that staff were more likely to report to work if shelter and family support issues such as child care and pet care were provided. Dosa et al. (2007) suggest that allowing staff families and pets to shelter at the facility will fix this problem. Then, off-duty staff can be identified to offer child and pet care for those on duty.

An alternative to the all-or-nothing evacuation approach is a more graduated methodology suggested by Dosa's group (Aldrich and Benson 2008). With this approach, the decision of whether or not to evacuate is based upon the summation of the assessed risks for the individual resident, the facility, and the event leading to an aggregate risk assessment. The event risk is the perceived danger of the particular hurricane—a Category 1 storm has little risk, a Category 3 storm has moderate risk, and a Category 5 storm is potentially cataclysmic. The facility risk is determined by the proximity of the facility to storm surge and the "hardness" of the physical plant. A poorly constructed, older nursing home on a flood plain within 1 mile of the ocean is at far higher facility risk than a new, hurricane-hardened facility 20 miles inland and 40 feet above sea level. Finally, the person risk is determined by the level of risk the evacuation engenders for a specific elderly resident. Elders with special medical needs, like dialysis or chronic oxygen therapy, and those with significant medical comorbidities, like congestive heart failure, would be scored higher risk than those more robust elders without such health challenges.

Once these risks have been assessed, the facility administrator and staff can choose to evacuate early those patients at higher risk if the event is significant and the facility is relatively at risk from the hurricane. Similarly, they could choose to hold off evacuating those more robust residents until later to see if the storm might miss the facility. Using this graduated approach makes intuitive sense, but more research is needed to see whether it actually improves outcomes.

Whether or not a specific residential care facility chooses to evacuate, every facility should have a disaster plan that is practical and easy to implement. A generic disaster plan for a nursing home that survived Hurricane Andrew in August 1992 was published in 1995 (Silverman et al. 1995). Some points to note about this plan include:

- The transportation plan should be addressed because local vendors probably will not suffice as noted previously (Dosa et al. 2007).

- The chain of command mentioned should be the IMS structure previously discussed (McCann 2009a; 2009b).

- The hurricane alert simulations ought to be full disaster drills that ideally would include buses and coordination with the presumed site of evacuation.

- Third-party vendor agreements and suppliers can be "verified annually," but if every other facility in the evacuation zone uses the same vendors, it is likely the facility's contracts may not be honored when a hurricane occurs.

- Vehicle and generator fuel should be stockpiled as it is likely that gas/diesel delivery to local vendors will be disrupted for days or weeks post-event.

- Cash-on-hand should involve significant funds as banks and ATMs may be nonfunctional for weeks or months.

- Waste management planning can be a significant burden for a residential care facility.

- The importance of coordinating the facility's plan with local and state officials and EOCs cannot be overemphasized (Dosa et al. 2008).

Dialysis-Dependent Elders

As noted previously, elders with special medical needs require careful disaster planning. This is especially true for those elders on dialysis. Major hurricanes can wreak havoc on dialysis facilities, rendering them nonfunctional for months after landfall. For instance, Hurricane Katrina precipitated the closure of 43 Louisiana dialysis facilities on August 31, 2005, and by December 31 half of these shuttered facilities had still not reopened (Network Coordinating Council 2005). There are over 300,000 dialysis-dependent patients in the United States (roughly one in 1,000 patients), so the prolonged loss of a significant number of dialysis facilities places a major strain on regional healthcare resources (USRDS 2006). Undamaged Louisiana dialysis facilities faced a tremendous surge of patients in the days after Hurricane Katrina. For example, the Renal Care Group facility in Baton Rouge usually cared for a census of 62 patients, but in the three days after Katrina, they dialyzed an additional 199 patients (Cary and Schroeder 2008)—an impressive feat since each hemodialysis procedure lasts four hours.

Elderly dialysis patients face numerous challenges after a hurricane—lack of transportation, lack of shelter, lack of appropriate food (a renal diet low in potassium and relatively fluid restricted), lack of routine medical care, lack of medications, and lack of availability of dialysis. When renal patients miss their dialysis for more than three days, they can rapidly decline and suffer complications such as uremia, hyperkalemia, and volume overload (Zoraster, Vanholder, and Sever 2007), ultimately resulting in death. The priority for these patients is clearly evacuation to facilities where dialysis can be provided, preferably well in advance of the storm. There are organizations that track availability of dialysis facilities such as the National Kidney Foundation (www.kidney.org), End Stage Renal Disease Networks (www.esrdnetworks.org), the American Society of Nephrology (www.asn-online.org), and the International Society of Nephrology (www.nature.com/isn/index.html) (Zoraster, Vanholder, and Sever 2007).

Unfortunately, post-hurricane circumstances often arise that prevent evacuation (flooding, washed-out roads, lack of transportation, etc.). When it is not feasible for renal patients to evacuate quickly, there are management methods that can help temporize for several days until evacuation is available (Zoraster, Vanholder, and Sever 2007):

1. Renal patients should limit dietary sodium intake to less than 65 mEq and potassium intake to less than 40 mEq daily. This means not using added salt or salt substitutes at meals as well as choosing foods that are low in sodium and potassium. In the latter case, high potassium foods such as fruits, vegetables, and chocolate must be avoided.

2. They should limit water intake to 500 cc a day and chew gum to help with thirst.

3. They should not fast; instead, frequent small carbohydrate-enriched meals are preferred. Shelters that may need to care for dialysis patients must have appropriate renal diet supplies on hand.

4. They should avoid constipation, which can be a risk factor for hyper-kalemia. Using laxatives as required is necessary. However, they should not use bran because it usually has a high potassium content.

5. They should carry a medication list at all times and have a substantial back-up supply of medications on hand.

6. Those on peritoneal dialysis should keep at least a week's worth of backup dialysate on hand. Peritoneal dialysis patients should know their usual body weight.

7. Those patients on hemodialysis should know their target post-dialysis weight.

As a result of the dialysis difficulties caused by Hurricanes Katrina and Rita, a strong collaborative network was formed in 2006—the Kidney Community Emergency Response Coalition (KCERC)—which involved nephrology associations, other chronic renal failure organizations, and government entities such as the National Institutes of Health, the Department of Health & Human Services, and the Food and Drug Administration. It included representatives from 25 states and the District of Columbia (Cary and Schroeder 2008). The purpose of KCERC's creation was to:

- help create a common, shared plan for national strategic disaster responses for the dialysis community,
- define clear roles and responsibilities to aid in the creation of such a plan,
- help disseminate best practices and strategies at both the state and local levels.
- To achieve these ends, nine separate response teams were created in the areas of:
- patient assistance,
- communications,

- patient tracking (always a major challenge post-disaster),
- dialysis facility operations,
- federal response,
- vendor services,
- leadership,
- planning and administration,
- pandemic planning.

The KCERC has been active in the years since Katrina helping to raise public awareness, promote the use of available tools, and further refining the nascent national strategy. This kind of collaborative effort is precisely what disaster planners need to do to ameliorate disaster response. It should be used as a model for disaster planning for the elderly in general.

POLICY RECOMMENDATIONS

This paper has considered the importance of improving disaster planning for the elderly, especially the frail, those in residential care, and those who are dialysis dependent. The literature in this regard is clear—the needs of the elderly before, during, and after hurricanes have not been adequately addressed or planned for during previous disasters. The following recommendations require urgent consideration to prevent another hurricane debacle like Katrina:

1. Local, state, and federal disaster planners must partner with aging services networks to improve access to elderly clients—such partnerships will contribute to decreased morbidity and mortality during hurricane disasters. These partnerships must remember that the elderly are an inhomogeneous cohort with widely varying needs. A perfect example of such a collaborative network is the KCERC for dialysis units.

2. Networks partnering with officials in this way must be familiar with the IMS and understand their role within it.

3. There is an urgent need for an effective surveillance tool, preferably

coupled with Global Information System (GIS) mapping, to determine the elderly population's likely needs during a hurricane. In particular, those with chronic diseases will need to be identified and required resources will need to be determined to allow their medical care post-disaster. This information must be shared with EOC planning personnel so that it can be incorporated into disaster planning.

4. Nursing homes and other elderly residential care facilities must have their disaster plans integrated into local, state, and federal disaster response plans. These plans must be exercised regularly in coordination with the local EOC.

5. Disaster planners, especially public health officials, must seek new and better ways to communicate principles of effective hurricane preparedness to the elderly, especially those with disabilities such as visual and hearing impairments. Community outreach through Public Health Departments would likely be an efficient means to achieve this.

6. Effective communication (including redundant forms of communication such as satellite phones, ham radio operators, etc.) is pivotal to disaster response and should be improved, especially between EOCs and residential care facilities.

7. Residential care facilities must be given the same priority access to return of essential services as hospitals.

8. Nursing homes must have a minimum of seven days worth of medical supplies, medication, and medical equipment as well as two weeks of food and water for all those sheltering at the facility (not just the elderly residents but also staff and the patient's family members).

9. Evacuation planning should be graduated rather than all-or-none and detailed evacuation plans should be available and tested regularly.

THE ROAD FORWARD

Given the apparent lack of disaster planning for the elderly in hurricane-prone coastal areas, it will be important for state and local EOCs to partner with elder advocacy groups to rectify this situation. At the federal level, the Assistant Secretary for Preparedness and Response in the Department of Health and Human Services should appoint a high-level advisor specifically tasked to consult with state governments, the American Association of Retired Persons (AARP), and other key stakeholders to improve elder hurricane preparedness. However, the most important first step is for the public sector to admit there is a major problem with disaster planning for the elderly and develop the political will to solve it before another mega storm like Katrina needlessly destroys lives.

REFERENCES

Aldrich, N., and W.F. Benson. 2008. "Disaster Preparedness and the Chronic Disease Needs of Vulnerable Older Adults." *Preventing Chronic Disease* 5 (1): 1-7.

Alson, R., D. Alexander, R.B. Leonard, and L.W. Stringer. 1193. "Analysis of Medical Treatment at a Field Hospital Following Hurricane Andrew, 1992." *Annals of Emergency* 22 (11): 1721-1728.

Auf der Heide, E. 2000. "CHAPTER 10—Principles of Disaster Planning." In *Disaster Preparedness in Schools of Public Health: A Curriculum for the New Century*, ed. L.Y. Landesman. New York. Association of Schools of Public Health.

Cary, S., and K. Schroeder. 2008. "Caring for Patients on Kidney Dialysis in a Disaster: Lessons from Baton Rouge after Hurricane Katrina." *American Journal of Nursing* 108 (1): 26-32.

Castro, C., D. Persson, N. Bergstrom, et al. 2008. "Surviving the Storms: Emergency Preparedness in Texas Nursing Facilities and Assisted Living Facilities." *Journal of Gerontological Nursing* 34 (8): 9-16.

Centers for Disease Control and Prevention. 2005. Update on CDC's Response to Hurricane Katrina [Internet]. Atlanta, GA: Centers for Disease Control and Prevention. http://www.cdc.gov/od/katrina/09-19-05.htm (accessed September 19).

Cherniack, E.P., L. Sandals, L. Brooks, et al. 2008. "Trial of a Survey Instrument to Establish the Hurricane Preparedness of and Medical Impact on a Vulnerable, Older Population." *Prehospital and Disaster Medicine* 23 (3): 242-249.

Dosa, D.M., K. Hyer, L.M. Brown, et al. 2008. "The Controversy Inherent in Managing Frail Nursing Home Residents During Complex Hurricane Emergencies." *Journal of the American Medical Directors Association* 9 (8): 599-604.

Dosa, D.M., N. Grossman, T. Wetle, et al. 2007. "To Evacuate or Not to Evacuate: Lessons Learned from Louisiana Nursing Home Administrators Following Hurricanes Katrina and Rita." *Journal of the American Medical Directors Association* 8: 142-149.

Dynes, R.R., E.L. Quarantelli, and G.A. Kreps. 1981. *A Perspective on Disaster Planning*, Third Edition. Newark, DE: Disaster Research Center, University of Delaware.

Federal Emergency Management Agency (FEMA) Emergency Management Institute IS-100 course. http://emilms.fema.gov/IS100b/ICS01 summary.htm.

Fernandez, L.S., D. Byard, C. Lin, et al. 2002. "Frail Elderly as Disaster Victims: Emergency Management Strategies." *Prehospital Disaster Medicine* 17 (2): 67-74.

Ford, E.S., A.H. Mokdad, M.W. Link, et al. 2006. "Chronic Diseases in Health Emergencies: In the Eye of the Hurricane." *Preventing Chronic Disease* 3 (2): 1-7. http://www.cdc.gov/pcd/issues/2006/apr/05_0235.htm.

Gibson, M.J. 2006. *We Can Do Better: Lessons Learned for Protecting Older Persons in Disasters*. Washington, DC: AARP. http://assets.aarp.org/rgcenter/il/better.pdf.

Gillick, M.R. 1994. *Choosing Medical Care in Old Age: What Kind, How Much, When to Stop*. Cambridge, MA: Harvard University Press. http://www.cdc.gov/aging/pdf/State_of_Aging_and_Health_in_America_2004.pdf.

Huxhold, O., S. Li, F. Schimiedek, et al. 2006. "Dual-Tasking Postural Control: Aging and Effects on Cognitive Demand in Conjunction with Focus on Attention." *Brain Research Bulletin* 69: 294-305.

Kilijanek, T.S., and T.E. Drabek. 1979. "Assessing Long-Term Impacts of a Natural Disaster: A Focus on the Elderly." *The Gerontologist* 19 (6): 555-566.

Laditka, S.B., J.N. Laditka, C.B. Cornman, et al. 2009. "Resilience and Challenges Among Staff of Gulf Coast Nursing Homes Sheltering Frail Evacuees Following Hurricane Katrina 2005: Implications for Planning and Training." *Prehospital Disaster Medicine* 24 (1): 54-62.

McCann, D.G.C. 2009a. "Disaster Medicine: A New Medical Specialty Comes of Age." *Forensic Sciences* 3 (3II): 1-79.

McCann, D.G.C. 2009b. "Preparing for the Worst: A Disaster Medicine Primer for Health Care." *Journal of Legal Medicine* 30: 329-348.

Mokdad, A.H., G.A. Mensah, S.F. Posner, et al. 2005. "When Chronic Conditions Become Acute: Prevention and Control of Chronic Diseases and Adverse Health Outcomes During Natural Disasters." *Preventing Chronic Disease* 2 (special issue). http://www.cdc.gov/pcd/issues/2005/nov/05_0201.htm.

Murphy, C., C.R. Schubert, K.J. Cruikshanks, et al. 2002. "Prevalence of Olfactory Impairments in Older Adults." *JAMA* 288: 2307-2312.

Nelson, D.E., D. Holtzman, J. Bolen, et al. 2001. "Reliability and Validity of Measures from the Behavioural Risk Factor Surveillance System (BRFSS)." *Soz Praventivmed* 46 (1): S3-S42.

Network Coordinating Council. End Stage Renal Disease Network 13. 2005. *2005 Annual Report*. Appendix G. Network Disaster Activities 2005: Hurricanes Katrina and Rita: Information Management. Oklahoma City, OK. http://www.network13.org/Data_Reports/Annual_Reports/2005/NW13_A R_2005.pdf.

Oriol, W. 1999. *Psychosocial Issues for Older Adults in Disasters*. Washington, DC: US Department of Health and Human Services, Substance Abuse and Mental Health Services Administration, Center for Mental Health Services.

Polivka-West, L., and A. Berman. 2008. "Safeguarding Seniors During Hurricanes: A New Report Highlights Steps All Nursing Homes Should Take." *American Journal of Nursing* 108 (1): 28-28.

Schoenborn, C.A., J.L. Vickerie, E. Powell-Griner, et al. 2006. "Health Characteristics of Adults 55 Years of Age and Older: United States, 2000–2003." *Advanced Data from Vital and Health Statistics* 370: 1-32.

Shatz, D.V., K. Wolcott, and J.B. Fairburn. 2006. "Response to Hurricane Disasters." *Surgical Clinics of North America* 86: 545-555.

Silverman, M.A., M. Weston, M. Llorente, C. Beber, and R. Tam. 1995. "Lessons Learned From Hurricane Andrew: Recommendations for Care of the Elderly in Long-term Care Facilities." *Southern Medical Journal* 88 (6): 603-608.

The State of Aging and Health in America 2004. 2004. Merck Institute of Aging and Health. US Department of Health and Human Services, Centers for Disease Control and Prevention. Atlanta, GA.

Townsend, F.F., et al. 2006. *The Federal Response to Hurricane Katrina: Lessons Learned.* The White House. Washington, DC. http://georgewbushwhitehouse.archives.gov/reports/katrina-lessons-learned.pdf.

US Renal Data System: USRDS 2006 Annual Data Report: Atlas of End Stage Renal Disease in the United States. http://www.usrds.org/adr.htm.

Zoraster, R., R. Vanholder, and M.S. Sever. 2007. "Disaster Management of Chronic Dialysis Patients." *American Journal of Disaster Medicine* 2 (2): 96-103.

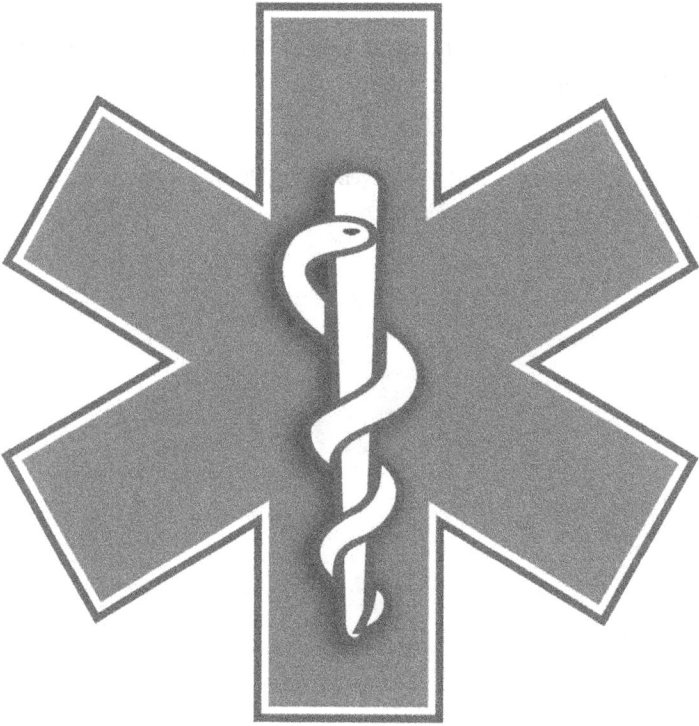

THE PUBLIC HEALTH IMPLICATIONS
OF WATER IN DISASTERS

David GC McCann, *McMaster University*
Ainsley Moore, *McMaster University*
Mary-Elizabeth A. Walker

INTRODUCTION

Water, water everywhere, and all the boards did shrink;
water, water everywhere, nor any drop to drink.

—*The Rime of the Ancient Mariner*, Samuel Taylor Coleridge

The World Health Organization (WHO) defines a disaster as "a serious disruption of the functioning of a community or a society causing widespread human, material, economic or environmental losses which exceed the ability of the affected community or society to cope using its own resources" (WHO 1998). The global incidence of disasters is increasing (Nicogossian et al. 2011) and water-related emergencies account for 40–50% of all disasters and disaster-related deaths (Du et al. 2010). The social determinants of health play a major role in water-related disasters because the poor (Paul and Routray 2010), the uneducated (Paul and Routray 2010), women (Nahar et al. 2010), the elderly (Cherniack 2008; McCann 2011), the very young (Kistin et al. 2010), and the disabled (Peek and Stough 2010) are more vulnerable.

Disasters may be natural (e.g. hurricanes) or related to human activity (e.g. terrorism). They can also be described as rapid onset (e.g. earthquakes and tsunamis) or slow onset (e.g. drought). Rapid onset disasters usually cause the majority of morbidity and mortality immediately while the slower onset type are more likely to cause harm through longer term, secondary effects (Murthy and Christian 2010).

Disaster Medicine is a new medical specialty that not only treats disaster victims but also deals with the medical issues related to disaster preparedness, mitigation, management, and recovery; the United States formally recognized the new medical specialty by executive order in 2007 (McCann 2009)

The American Board of Disaster Medicine (ABODM) is the world's first physician board of certification in the nascent specialty. ABODM's sister organization, the American Academy of Disaster Medicine (AADM), acts as the academic arm of the new specialty, promoting research into best practices and collaboration among public and private sector partners. As the new discipline matures, developing a coordinated, standardized international approach to disasters, especially in developing countries that struggle with response to water-related disasters, will be a major policy priority (McCann and Cordi 2011).

Whether a disaster involves too little water (e.g. drought), water excess (e.g. floods and tsunamis), or water contamination during or after the event, there is an inextricable connection among disasters, water, and public health. In the immediate and long-term post-disaster periods, water, food, and shelter become either critical lifesaving or hazardous resources depending upon how they are utilized. This paper examines the most current literature in this subject area and offers perspectives for policymakers to improve water security.

WATER SHORTAGE—DROUGHT

Drought develops slowly over a period of months to years and is caused by lower than average precipitation in a given area over an extended timeframe, leading to an inadequate supply of water. Approximately 15% of the world's natural disasters are caused by drought and drought-related deaths account for 59% of the world's extreme weather mortalities (Raphael et al. 2009). Multiple authors have linked climate change to drought severity, although a definitive cause-and-effect relationship remains inconclusive (Kistin et al. 2010; Raphael et al. 2009; Ebi, Helmer, and Vainio 2008; Friel et al. 2011; Horton, Hanna, and Kelly 2010; Saniotis and Bi 2009). There are significant public health implications related to drought; public health staff and other health professionals require evidence-based recommendations for dealing with the health consequences of water shortage. A multi-agency collaboration in the United States recently developed such recommendations which are an important addition to the literature (Centers for Disease Control and Prevention 2010).

Water is required for food production. To produce one calorie of plant food at least one liter of water is required, while one calorie of meat or dairy food production utilizes up to 10 liters of water (Wahlquist 2009). Thus, drought frequently results in decreased food production. Parts of Australia, for example, have suffered from drought for three decades, which has adversely impacted much of the continent. Drought has been especially problematic in the Murray-Darling Basin, the agricultural heartland of Australia, resulting in a significant diminution in its crop and livestock output (Wahlquist 2009). Recently, China, too, has suffered drought in some of its provinces including Yunnan, Sichuan, Guizhou, and Chongqing, causing delayed crop planting and livestock failure to thrive (Chan and Griffiths 2010). Even without drought, China's water resources are scarce; they have only 7% of the world's freshwater but support 20% of the world's population with significant regional disparities in water supply (Zhang et al. 2010).

Severe drought can eventually lead to famine as has occurred frequently in Ethiopia (Taye, Mariam, and Murray 2010). It can cause significant population displacement as well (Friel et al. 2011). Note that children are particularly at an increased risk of adverse health effects, especially when drought results in famine and malnutrition

(Kistin et al. 2010). The elderly, too, are more susceptible to the negative physical health effects of drought (Horton, Hanna, and Kelly 2010; Saniotis and Bi 2009).

In addition to lack of potable water, drought causes negative effects on air quality because of prolonged particulate suspension in the air column. Increased airborne particulates negatively impact human lung function, especially in people with chronic lung diseases like asthma (Kalis and Wilson 2009). Wildfires are more common in drought-stricken areas and the smoke from these fires also contributes to deranged lung function (Kalis and Wilson 2009). Recreational water activities can become hazardous as a result of increased pollution of surface water (Kalis and Wilson 2009). Vector-borne diseases may proliferate. For instance, water shortage leads to mosquitoes breeding in atypical areas nearer to birds and other wildlife. The result can be outbreaks of St. Louis encephalitis, eastern equine encephalitis (Kalis and Wilson 2009), and West Nile virus (Wang et al. 2010). There can also be increased incidence of other diseases such as the fungal disease coccidioidomycosis, the spores of which are increasingly aerosolized by drought conditions, making them easier to inhale (Kalis and Wilson 2009).

Drought can also negatively impact mental health. The main psychosocial effects include poor quality of life, significantly altered lifestyle, and conflict over insufficient water resources (Keim 2008). Australia's drought has taken a significant mental health toll on adolescents (Dean and Stain 2010), the elderly, and rural area residents, especially farmers (Horton, Hanna, and Kelly 2010). A study in New South Wales demonstrated that over half the population surveyed felt that drought was extremely or very likely to continue; 60.1% were extremely concerned about the effect of drought on them; and as a result 86.3% had made some changes in the way they lived. Such perceptions are inherently stressful and could have negative repercussions on mental health. These attitudes were especially prevalent among women, those living in rural areas, and families with children under 16 years of age. Interestingly, respondents over 55 years were less inclined to feel drought was highly likely to continue, perhaps related to their broader life experience (Raphael et al. 2009).

EXCESS WATER—FLOODS AND TSUNAMIS

Floods are the most common type of disaster worldwide. Storm surges are the most dangerous aspect of hurricanes as people along the Mississippi coastline discovered during the landfall of Hurricane Katrina. Tsunamis are one of nature's most awesome spectacles; in fact, a tsunami may have accounted for Plato's legendary lost city of Atlantis (Llewellyn 2006). What these various types of events have in common is an excess of water; what varies among them is the speed with which that excess occurs.

FLOODS AND STORM SURGES

Floods occur either by bodies of water overflowing their banks or by water accumulating in low-lying areas (Du et al. 2010). In the United States, for example, floods account for approximately 90% of natural disaster damage when droughts are excluded. The cost of U.S. floods between 1988 and 1997 averaged $3.7 billion dollars annually (Llewellyn 2006). In developing countries, the human cost of floods is much greater, especially in terms of lives lost and populations displaced. In the 2007 Bangladesh flood, for instance, over 7.5 million people were affected with 250,000 seeking refuge in temporary shelters (Nahar et al. 2010).

Floods can develop slowly, such as in northern latitudes when winter snows melt and ice-choked rivers crest above flood stage over a period of days to weeks (riverine floods). On the other hand, "flash floods" can develop over a period of several hours, either from sudden heavy precipitation or dam/reservoir/levee breach. It was the breach of the 17th Street levee in New Orleans after Hurricane Katrina that inundated the Lower 9th Ward (Du et al. 2010). Flash floods cause the majority of drowning deaths, usually because victims underestimate the strength of the current and the depth of the water. According to the Red Cross, "six inches of swiftly moving water can sweep you off your feet" (Red Cross 2009). In developed countries, the majority of flood deaths occur in motor vehicles when drivers inappropriately try to navigate flooded roads and bridges or crash due to poor driving conditions. In the United States, more than 57% of flood mortality is automobile-related (Du et al. 2010). The Red Cross asserts that only two feet of moving water is required to sweep vehicles away (Red Cross 2009). Fortunately, improved meteorological forecasting has decreased flash flood mortality by >50% (Keim 2008).

Floods have both direct and indirect health effects. The most immediate effect is drowning. Those who do not drown may sustain orthopedic and soft tissue injuries from floating debris, electrical injuries from downed power lines, burns and trauma related to gas leaks and ruptured chemical tanks, hypothermia, and loss of health services (e.g. hospitals and clinics) in the flooded area. Secondary health effects of flooding include water contamination (discussed later), carbon monoxide poisoning from inappropriately located gas-powered generators, and increased respiratory illnesses related to mold exposure and microbial growth (Du et al. 2010). After Hurricanes Katrina and Rita, the burden of fungal spores in flooded houses was significantly elevated with Aspergillus niger, Penicillium sp., Trichoderma, and Paecilomyces, all of which can cause either respiratory or dermatological disease, particularly in individuals who are immunocompromised (Murthy and Christian 2010).

Outbreaks of diarrheal illness have occurred after some floods but are not as common as might be expected. Common pathogens associated with post-disaster diarrheal outbreaks include cholera, Giardia, Shigella, Salmonella, and various viral illnesses such as rotavirus and norovirus (Murthy and Christian 2010), When diarrheal outbreaks occur, they are usually caused by pathogens that already existed in the local environment pre-flood, such as Shigella and Giardia; however, in most cases a specific cause is never determined and drinking water is merely assumed to be the source (Murthy and Christian 2010). For instance, there was a waterborne outbreak of cholera after Cyclone Aila in India in 2009 that lasted from

May through August of that year. This was not surprising because cholera is endemic in India. This particular epidemic was eventually controlled through repairing broken water pipelines, chlorination of household drinking water, and through public education (Bhunia and Ghosh 2011). In the month of August 2007, Bangladesh's Dhaka Hospital treated 21,401 cases of diarrheal illness as a result of severe flooding, more than three times the amount treated in the same month in 2006 (Nahar et al. 2010).

Overall, communicable diseases are less common after floods than after other types of disasters. When they do occur, they tend to be related to overcrowded shelters, poor personal hygiene, lack of clean water, poor sanitation, poor nutrition, and increases in disease-carrying vectors like mosquitoes (Du et al. 2010; Murthy and Christian 2010). For example, a powerful cyclone, Sidr, hit Bangladesh in 2007 and did significant damage. Once again, authorities feared epidemics of water-borne, respiratory, and other diseases, but the dire predictions never materialized. In fact, a study demonstrated the illness prevalence to be only 3.6% after Sidr largely due to early distribution of food and water, proper medical care, and effective public health interventions (Paul and Routray 2010). Of course, there are exceptions, such as the previously mentioned diarrheal outbreak in Bangladesh's Dhaka Hospital.

The mental health effects of floods can be long term and debilitating. Flood victims are four times more likely to suffer psychological distress compared with people who have not suffered a flood. Flood victims are also 13.8% more likely to commit suicide after flooding compared to pre-flood (Du et al. 2010). A study of the mental health issues of children who survived Hurricane Katrina in 2005 demonstrated that 29% of pediatric primary care visits between July 2007 and June 2009 involved mental health issues or developmental and learning problems that required significant case intervention. The majority of these children showed disruptive behavior associated with underlying mood or anxiety disorders, but many of them had demonstrated pre-existing mental health challenges (Olteanu et al. 2011). Another study involving youth post-Katrina found similar results.

At baseline examination between 18 and 27 months after Katrina, 15.1% of youth showed signs of mental health disorders. On follow-up 12–18 months later (30–45 months after the storm), 11.2% of youth still demonstrated psychiatric problems, compared with only a 4.2% prevalence of psychiatric disturbance before Katrina (McLaughlin et al. 2010). In contradistinction, some studies described in a recent review article found the elderly may be more psychologically resilient in floods because they had been exposed to similar circumstances before (Cherniack 2008).

In the United Kingdom (UK), a cross-sectional survey of 444 flood victims found that 27.9% suffered from post-traumatic stress disorder (PTSD) symptoms, 24.5% from anxiety, and 35.1% from depression, with women showing more symptoms on average than men. Factors associated with greater psychological distress included displacement, poor health, and previous flood experiences (Mason, Andrews, and Upton 2010). This latter finding differed from another UK group who found prior exposure to flooding increased individual preparedness (Coulston and Deeny 2010).

In Bangladesh, a study of flood-related mental health effects found that higher household income and better employment predicted better access to food and water, resulting in better coping post-flood. Similarly, higher educational achievement allowed better access to pre-flood warnings, decreasing vulnerability, and increasing coping capacity. However, prolonged flooding with higher water levels and household location in closer proximity to riverbanks caused increased external stressors and decreased coping post-flood (Paul and Routray 2010).

Whereas floods can result from a variety of weather conditions, storm surges are caused by hurricane-force winds and the low-pressure induced vacuum effect of a tropical cyclone. The size of the storm surge depends to a significant degree on the shape of the coastline, the slope of the sea floor, and the stage of the tidal cycle when the storm hits. The majority of cyclone-associated mortality is caused by the storm surge (Murthy and Christian 2010). For instance, Hurricane Katrina's storm surge reached

27 feet in parts of Mississippi and leveled structures along the coastline for up to several miles inland (Centers for Disease Control and Prevention 2006), while the surge from Hurricane Camille in 1969 reached 25 feet and similarly decimated the Gulf Coast (Llewellyn 2006). Although the public had several days warning to evacuate in advance of Katrina, a significant number of residents chose to "ride it out." Many of those who remained along the Mississippi coast where the storm surge was the worst were swept away and drowned—a typical "rapid onset disaster" despite the advance warning. The post-disaster health effects of storm surge are basically the same as other floods (Murthy and Christian 2010).

TSUNAMIS

The Japanese translation of tsunami means "harbor wave." Tsunamis are caused by underwater earthquakes, volcanoes, or landslides that displace huge amounts of seawater, creating waves that can pummel coastal regions; since 1850, more than 400,000 people have been killed by these enormous "walls of water" (Llewellyn 2006).

The March 2011 moment magnitude 9.0 earthquake and the resulting tsunami in northeast Japan riveted the world's attention for weeks after the event (Normile 2011), in part because of the damage sustained at the Fukushima Daiichi Nuclear Power Plant and the release of a significant amount of radiation into the environment (Matsumoto and Inoue 2011). As this analysis is written, there is no end in sight for the worst nuclear power disaster since Chernobyl. The death toll from the earthquake and tsunami currently exceeds 28,000, although an accurate total will likely never be known since thousands of victims were simply washed out to sea (UN OCHA 2011).

The worst tsunami in recorded history occurred in late December 2004 after a moment magnitude 9.3 earthquake off the island of Sumatra—the Andaman-Nicobar earthquake and tsunami. This singular event resulted in more than 220,000 killed or missing in more than a dozen countries throughout the Indian Ocean Region (Guha-Sapir and van

Panhuis 2009). People in the westernmost part of Indonesia, the worst hit area, witnessed a giant wave of black water 50–80 feet high (Morrow and Llewellyn 2006). Aceh province lost nearly three-quarters of its population and more than half of all survivors were left homeless (Guha-Sapir and van Panhuis 2009). Unlike the extensive tsunami warning system in the Pacific Ocean, the Indian Ocean had no such early warning system in 2004. Thus, the coastal areas had no indication of the impending disaster.

A study of the health impacts of the 2004 tsunami in Aceh province examined the incidence of cholera, tetanus, wounds and wound infections, acute respiratory infections, malaria, and dengue pre- and post-event (Guha-Sapir and van Panhuis 2009). Widespread speculation held that communicable disease outbreaks would be problematic in the wake of the disaster, although previous literature did not support such claims (de Ville de Goyet 2007). In fact, the study found no confirmed cholera cases in the four months post-tsunami. The incidence of malaria and dengue, traditionally low compared with the rest of Indonesia, did not increase. Tetanus cases tripled in the weeks after the event with a peak reported during January 8–17, 2005. Nonetheless, there was no "epidemic of tetanus" (Rahardjo, Wiroatmodjo, and Koeshartono 2008). Traumatic injuries, including wounds, fractures, and general trauma, were significantly more common up to eight weeks after the tsunami but reduced to just a few by week 16. Multiple cases of aspiration pneumonia were reported and causal organisms tended to be highly unusual and resistant to common antibiotics (Guha-Sapir and van Panhuis, 2009). The unusual pathogens were likely related to the tsunami water containing organisms to which human populations would never normally be exposed.

The Andaman-Nicobar tsunami significantly impacted international tourist beach destinations like Phuket, Thailand. Victims from multiple European countries required emergency evacuation and treatment. A study conducted at three airport clinics in Europe set up to receive tsunami victims (Stockholm, Helsinki, and London) demonstrated psychological and physical illnesses, including soft tissue and orthopedic injuries, pneumothoraces, near-drowning, and aspiration pneumonias. As was found in the study previously mentioned (Guha-Sapir and van Panhuis 2009), the wound infections and pneumonias were often caused by bizarre and highly drug-resistant organisms as well as by methicillin-resistant Staphylococcus aureus (Deebaj et al. 2011).

Like other flood events, tsunamis can have long-term effects on the mental health of survivors. A study of 12,784 victims of the 2004 Andaman-Nicobar tsunami (Math et al. 2008) compared displaced and non-displaced victims and found a higher prevalence of psychiatric illness in the displaced but an equal distribution of depression and PTSD in both groups. Overall, 37.5% demonstrated adjustment disorder, 21.5% depression, 12% panic, 11.2% PTSD, and 5.5% anxiety. Factors that were found to be psychologically protective included:

- belonging to a cohesive community,
- good family system,
- good social support,
- altruistic behavior by community leaders,
- religious faith and spirituality

Some important lessons were learned from the 2004 tsunami disaster response (de Ville de Goyet 2008; 2007; Rahardjo, Wiroatmodjo, and Koeshartono 2008; von Schreeb et al. 2008):

- Tsunamis result in relatively few survivors—most victims die immediately by drowning. Only 10% of the wounded (approximately 7,200) in Aceh required hospitalization (von Schreeb et al. 2008).

- Foreign mobile hospitals deployed in the tsunami zone lacked coordination and many arrived too late to be of much use. By day 20, there were nine foreign mobile hospitals in operation but bed occupancy rates were <50%. The USNS Mercy Hospital Ship with 12 operating theaters and 1,000 beds arrived in Aceh from San Diego five weeks after the tsunami (Morrow and Llewellyn 2006; von Schreeb et al. 2008).

- Efficient use of existing local facilities proved more valuable than the foreign mobile facilities (Rahardjo, Wiroatmodjo, and Koeshartono 2008).

- Prognostication of epidemics was exaggerated.

- Re-establishment of water and sanitation should be the first priority.

- Excessive medical volunteerism actually did more harm than good, as there was no coordination of activities. Further, volunteer responders were often reluctant to share operational information with one another because of a competitive humanitarian environment.

- Foreign monetary aid was excessive (>$7000 US per affected person) and humanitarian aid groups vied aggressively for these dollars.

- Logistics of sorting through massive amounts of international donations overwhelmed local capacity and most of the perishables were lost. Some of the medical equipment and training offered by international groups was totally inappropriate for the Indonesian reality.

Undoubtedly, many lessons will be gleaned from the 2011 Japan earthquake and tsunami, but it seems likely that the Japanese will be more self-sufficient than countries in the developing world devastated by the 2004 tsunami. It will be interesting to see if Japan is capable of mounting a more streamlined, efficient response.

WATER CONTAMINATION

Water contamination is common after disasters. The human health effects of water contamination can compound the misery engendered by the disaster event and can sometimes continue for months or even years. Oil spills are an appropriate example of the effect water contamination can have on human populations.

OIL SPILLS

Fossil fuels are an important part of modern life but their use can have significant negative effects on the environment and human health, particularly when oil spillage occurs. The explosion of the Deepwater Horizon drilling platform off the Louisiana coast in 2010 caused the catastrophic release of 800 million liters of oil into the Gulf of Mexico. This event will have long-term effects on the economy and health of Gulf Coast residents that are only now beginning to be appreciated (McCauley 2010; Diaz 2011). In fact, there have been at least 38 oil accidents in the last 50 years, 20 of which have been major spills (McCauley 2010).

Studies on the human health effects of oil spills have been few and usually cross-sectional. A recent review of these studies by Aguilera et al. (2010) found that human health effects of exposure to oil spills tended to be short-lived and reversible, including headaches, throat, and eye irritation. However, ingestion or aspiration of petroleum products can have serious health consequences, including acute chemical pneumonitis and neurological damage. The chemical constituents of oil and their various effects on human physiology are reviewed by Diaz (2011).

A study of workers involved in the cleanup of the 2003 Tasman Spirit oil spill in Karachi, Pakistan, found that 38% experienced cough, 36% a runny nose, 32% eye redness, 28% a sore throat, 28% headaches, 24% nausea, and 18% experienced "general illness" (Meo et al. 2009). Chung and Kim (2010) compared the physical and psychological symptoms of Korean survivors of a typhoon with those who lived in an area affected by an oil spill. Oil spill victims had more distressing physical and mental health effects than those who survived a typhoon. The authors suggested this was probably due to the toxic effects of oil on the body and the long-term, uncertain nature of oil spills compared with the short-term, self-limited effects of a typhoon. For the Deepwater Horizon Gulf oil spill, large amounts of the chemical dispersant Corexit 9500 were used and the possible long-term health effects related to this compound should also be considered (Diaz 2011).

Longer term health effects of oil spills are predominantly psychological and include increased generalized anxiety disorder, PTSD, and depression (Aguilera et al. 2010). Psychological effects are more pronounced in women, and, in the case of the Exxon Valdez Alaska oil spill of 1989, among the indigenous peoples. A study involving people affected by the 2002 Prestige oil spill off northwest Spain found community social support to be psychologically protective. Other protective factors included active participation in helping to solve the problem, and sufficient government economic aid to those affected (Sabucedo et al. 2010).

In vitro and animal toxicology studies noted induction of DNA damage by oil spill residues with metabolic enzymatic transformation of the fossil fuel compounds resulting in more toxic intermediaries (Aguilera et al. 2010). Other data suggest that short-term exposure to oil (5 days) causes reversible DNA damage whereas longer-term exposure (several months) results in irreversible DNA damage (McCauley 2010).

EARTHQUAKES

Large earthquakes can generate tsunamis as previously mentioned. However, earthquakes can also affect water quality in other ways, particularly through degradation of water and sanitation infrastructure. Diarrheal illnesses can be a significant source of morbidity and mortality after disasters like earthquakes, usually as a result of drinking water contamination (Magan et al. 2010).

An earthquake in the Kashmir region of the Indo-Pakistani border in October 2005 led to an outbreak of rotavirus diarrheal illness from October to December. The attack rate among children under five years of age was 20%. The rotavirus outbreak was traced to tap water obtained from groundwater sources that was stored and delivered untreated. This groundwater system had not caused diarrheal illness prior to the earthquake; after the earthquake, however, some refugee camps were set up near these groundwater sources. The conditions in these camps were suboptimal with significant overcrowding, poor sanitation, open-air defecation, and poor hygiene. Thus, the water supply became contaminated with fecal matter (Karmakar et al. 2008). This could have been avoided if adequate trench latrines had been provided to the camps in a timely fashion.

A study by Magan et al. (2010) after the same earthquake evaluated five densely populated urban centers that lacked proper access to potable water and sanitation prior to the disaster. The drinking water was derived from surface water contaminated with untreated wastewater and agricultural effluent. It was noted that even when water was properly treated at the source, it almost invariably became coliform contaminated in the piping system. Pipes often ran inside open waste and stormwater channels. Magan and coworkers recommended that adequate stockpiles of water treatment chemicals and storage containers be maintained as part of a water system emergency preparedness program. Other interventions for preventing future post-disaster diarrheal outbreaks include (Karmakar et al. 2008):

- Chlorine tablet distribution and public education about water chlorination.
- Public health water engineers should ensure water is adequately chlorinated by testing wells, storage tanks, etc. on a regular basis.
- Early provision of trench latrines to displaced persons to prevent open-air defecation and groundwater contamination.
- Promotion of hand washing with soap and water.

The January 2010 earthquake in Haiti caused catastrophic damage with 250,000 dead, 300,000 injured, and more than 1.3 million displaced (Walton and Ivers 2011). Even before the earthquake, Haiti's water and sanitation were practically nonexistent. Haiti ranked 147th out of 147 countries in water security in 2002 (Ivers et al. 2010). In 2008, only 63% of Haitians had access to safe water and 17% to adequate sanitation facilities. Diarrheal disease was a leading cause of child mortality before the Haitian earthquake as a result of contaminated water (Dowell, Tappero, and Frieden 2011), accounting for 16% of under age 5 childhood mortality (WHO 2010).

Haiti did not suffer a diarrheal epidemic until nine months after the earthquake when cholera struck the Artibonite basin, more than 55 miles from the nearest refugee camp. In mid-October, 60 cases of acute diarrhea were reported at a local hospital. Two days later the cause was confirmed to be cholera, which had not occurred in Haiti in more than a century. When Hurricane Tomas hit Haiti in November, it caused significant flooding that spread the cholera throughout the country. By the end of December, 2010, cholera had sickened more than 170,000 people and caused more than 3600 deaths (Dowell, Tappero, and Frieden 2011).

The specific cholera strain causing the Haitian epidemic was identified as Vibrio cholerae O1, serotype Ogawa, biotype El Tor, the DNA sequencing of which pointed to a Southeast Asian origin, possibly introduced by the United Nations Peacekeeping Force. This circumstance is a unique exception to the general principle that post-disaster diarrheal outbreaks involve pathogens that existed in the area prior to the disaster (Bhunia and Ghosh 2011). Unfortunately, the El Tor strain is notoriously more virulent, better able to survive in the environment, and more drug resistant than other cholera biotypes (Walton and Ivers 2011).

Over the last decade, multiple studies have found patterns of cholera spread relative to certain climatic and host factors. Remote sensing (RS) technology has played an important role in helping to delineate the climatic factors. A provocative time series analysis, published by Koelle and colleagues in Nature (2005), demonstrated that cholera's periodicity in Matlab, Bangladesh, over the last four decades is related to the timing of monsoon rains, sea surface temperature in the Bay of Bengal, the el Nino effect, and to variations in host immunity in the affected area. Other authors have published similar findings from studies in various places around the world (Alajo, Nakavuma, and Erume 2006; Anyamba et al. 2006; Gavilan and Martinez-Urtaza 2011; Hashizume et al. 2011; Martinez-Urtaza et al. 2008; Ohtomo et al. 2010; Olago et al. 2007). In one field trial, using sari cloth at the point of use for water filtration decreased cholera cases by 50% compared with a control group (Colwell and Wilcox 2010; Huq et al. 2010). These findings may have important implications for understanding and controlling the Haiti cholera epidemic, particularly the use of RS technology for epidemiological surveillance.

Eradicating El Tor cholera from Haiti will be a major challenge. Concerted international action with Haitian public health authorities will be required in order to (Ivers et al. 2010):

- Stockpile and distribute cholera vaccine—with economies of scale the cost is estimated to be less than US $1 per dose for the "Shanchol" vaccine.

- Identify and treat all those infected with cholera with either oral or IV rehydration and antibiotics. Although antibiotics are not routinely recommended for cholera treatment, they are helpful in epidemic situations, decreasing the length of illness and bacterial shedding, which could be important in getting control of El Tor.

- Address Haiti's infrastructure for water and sanitation—make sure soap, treated water, and adequate latrines are available to all Haitians.

- Ensure that all vertical health projects (e.g. for AIDS, women's health, etc.) help strengthen Haiti's health system. Building capacity is critical to long-term success.

FLOODS, TSUNAMIS, AND STORM SURGES

As noted previously, drinking contaminated water after flood events can lead to diarrheal outbreaks, often due to E. coli, Shigella, and Salmonella. Hepatitis A viral outbreaks are also possible (Du et al. 2010). Boil water advisories are common when water contamination has occurred. However, a study after the Andaman-Nicobar tsunami found water boiling was not effective whereas obtaining water from improved sources (e.g. tube wells instead of surface water sources) and household water chlorination did prove effective

(Gupta et al. 2007). The authors suggested possible reasons for the ineffectiveness of water boiling which included inadequate boiling procedures, poor water handling procedures after boiling, and the possibility of false reporting of boiling. Other drinking water safety strategies include (Shimi et al. 2010):

- Having tube wells on raised bases that do not sink during flooding.

- Having a cement base on tube wells to prevent floodwater contamination.

- Raising the height of the well head with pipe to maintain it above flood level.

- Using water purification tablets or alum when chlorine is unavailable.

Flooding can also cause water contamination with chemical effluents from agriculture or industry. Farm runoff, for example, can result in significant coastal water algal blooms that adversely affect human health (Du et al. 2010). Casteel and coworkers (2006) demonstrated that flooding from Hurricane Floyd and other storms in North Carolina in 1999 caused floodwater contamination with human and animal sewage pathogens that could adversely affect crops and livestock by contamination of agricultural soils. Industrial chemical effects, on the other hand, vary depending on the nature and concentration of the pollutant in the water supply. Obviously, frequent water quality assessment after flooding is necessary to minimize health risk in either case. Geographic Information Systems (GIS) mapping is helpful in disaster situations for tracking water/sanitation system status, resident contact information, water treatment alerts, etc. (Englande 2008).

After tsunamis, water is frequently contaminated with Gram negative bacteria, including Vibrio cholerae, Vibrio parahemolyticus, Aeromonas, Plesiomonas (Kanungo et al. 2007), Klebsiella, and Proteus. Another post-tsunami study found other unusual pathogens, including Acinetobacter, Pseudomonas, Stenotrophomonas, E. coli, and Mucor, were common and difficult to treat (Murthy and Christian 2010). Wounds contaminated with these uncommon pathogens can become severely infected and may be treatment resistant. The experience after the Andaman-Nicobar tsunami suggests that such wounds be vigorously debrided, left open to heal by secondary intention (Prasartritha, Tungsiripat, and Warachit 2008), and treated with beta lactam penicillins. After three days of antibiotic therapy, if improvement is not noted, the patient should then be treated with ciprofloxacin or one of the newer quinolones, possibly in combination with gentamicin depending on the local experience with antibiotic resistance patterns (Okumura et al. 2009). Wound culture prior to institution of empirical antibiotic therapy is highly recommended.

SUMMARY AND POLICY RECOMMENDATIONS

Water security is an important aspect of disaster planning and recovery. This article makes it clear that much work needs to be done to improve sanitation and water systems globally, particularly in developing countries like Haiti. Unfortunately, billions of dollars in international aid frequently get diverted away from critical infrastructure improvement projects in favor of more immediate needs in the developing world. Such policies are myopic and counterproductive. The political and social will should be fostered to generate public health policies, which invest in long-term infrastructure improvements in water and sanitation, preventing much of the human misery compounded by disasters.

Examples of policies for improving water security in disaster situations are as follows:

1. Re-establish safe water and effective sanitation as a major priority in the immediate aftermath of an emergency. Adequate numbers of trench latrines will suffice to prevent open-air defecation that contaminates groundwater. Where bottled water is not available, household water chlorination is highly effective, more so than simply boiling water. Public education in proper chlorine treatment is essential.

2. Shelters must not be overcrowded and should have adequate latrines and safe water with plenty of hand washing stations and liquid soap available. Also, alcohol hand sanitizing solution deployment would be another effective method to promote decreased fecal oral transmission in shelters.

3. Public education on personal hygiene instituted in advance of a disaster and reinforced frequently.

4. Effective use of community groups and NGOs to spread important risk communication messages after disasters is important. Such organizations should work closely with government and public health officials to coordinate effective messaging to the public (e.g. how to chlorinate water).

5. Volunteerism can cause chaos in disaster situations. Volunteers must be coordinated and appropriately credentialed (especially health professionals) through a central volunteer coordination center (Englande 2008). "Disaster tourism" is strongly discouraged as it diverts essential supplies from those who need them to support "disaster tourists."

6. Vector control (e.g. spraying to kill mosquitoes) is important after a disaster to prevent epidemics of vector-borne illnesses like malaria and dengue. These vectors tend to propagate in stagnant water,

7. Post-disaster epidemics related to contaminated water are not as common as popularly believed. Appropriate disease surveillance and timely public health interventions can mitigate this risk significantly.

8. Effective mental health services must be available to victims of disaster in a timely fashion. As mentioned earlier, water-related disasters have potential long-term negative effects on survivor mental health. Responding to this need requires careful planning before an event to ensure availability of trained personnel in disaster areas.

9. Adequate stockpiles of water treatment chemicals and storage

containers need to be maintained as part of an overall emergency preparedness program. There should also be adequate stockpiles of vaccines including cholera, hepatitis A, and tetanus.

10. Public health engineers must ensure water treatment is effective by regularly testing wells, water storage tanks, etc. to ensure safety.

11. Redundancy in design of decentralized water and sanitation systems is important (Englande 2008). Capacity building for these critical infrastructures is important

12. GIS mapping is an important mechanism to track water and sanitation system status, water treatment alerts, resident contact information, etc. (Englande 2008). This valuable information is costly and is primarily used by developed countries and should be part of the humanitarian assistance package offered to developing countries through international collaborative efforts. Prior agreements on the use of this technology to ensure the confidentiality of the host country as well as its economic and military security should be achieved through such organizations as the United Nations.

In conclusion, the intersection of water and human health in disasters will continue to be an area of important research and public policy debate because disasters are becoming more common.

This review has summarized the most current knowledge in the area of water safety following disasters and derived policy recommendations based upon the best evidence available. This information should stimulate and motivate international cooperation toward improved capacity for safe water and sanitation globally. Effective international cooperation in developing best practices for recovery and response is an urgent priority (McCann and Cordi 2011).

REFERENCES

Aguilera, F., J. Mendez, E. Pasaro, and B. Laffon. 2010. "Review on the Effects of Exposure to Spilled Oils on Human Health." *Journal of Applied Toxicology: JAT* 30 (4): 291-301.

Alajo, S. O., J. Nakavuma, and J. Erume. 2006. "Cholera in Endemic Districts in Uganda During El Nino Rains: 2002-2003." *African Health Sciences* 6 (2): 93-97.

Anyamba, A., J. P. Chretien, J. Small, C. J. Tucker, and K. J. Linthicum. 2006. "Developing Global Climate Anomalies Suggest Potential Disease Risks for 2006-2007." *International Journal of Health Geographics* 5: 60.

Bhunia, R., and S. Ghosh. 2011. "Waterborne Cholera Outbreak Following Cyclone Aila in Sundarban Area of West Bengal, India, 2009." *Transactions of the Royal Society of Tropical Medicine and Hygiene* 105 (4): 214-219.

Casteel MJ, Sobsey MD, Mueller JP 2006. "Fecal contamination of agricultural soils before and after hurricane-associated flooding in North Carolina." *J Environ Sci Health A Tox Hazard Subst Environ Eng.* 41(2):173-84.

Centers for Disease Control and Prevention, US Environmental Protection Agency, National Oceanic and Atmospheric Agency, American Water Works Association. 2006. "Rapid Community Needs Assessment after Hurricane Katrina—Hancock County, Mississippi, September 14-15, 2005." *MMWR. Morbidity and Mortality Weekly Report* 55 (9): 234-236.

Centers for Disease Control and Prevention, U.S. Environmental Protection Agency, National Oceanic and Atmospheric Agency and American Water Works Association. 2010. "When every drop counts: protecting public health during drought conditions — a guide for public health officials." Atlanta: U.S. Department of Health and Human Services. Available at www.cdc.gov/nceh/ehs/Docs/When_Every_Drop_Counts.pdf

Chan, E., and S. Griffiths. 2010. "The Implication of Water on Public Health: The Case of China." *Perspectives in Public Health* 130 (5): 209-210.

Cherniack, E.P. 2008. "The Impact of Natural Disasters on the Elderly." *American Journal of Disaster Medicine* 3 (3): 133-139.

Chung S and E. Kim. 2010. Physical and mental health of disaster victims: a comparative study on typhoon and oil spill disasters. *J Prev Med Public Health.* 2010 Sep;43(5):387-95.

Colwell, R.R., and B.A. Wilcox. 2010. "Water, Ecology, and Health." *EcoHealth* 7 (2): 151-152.

Coulston, J.E., and P. Deeny. 2010. "Prior Exposure to Major Flooding Increases Individual Preparedness in High-risk Populations." *Prehospital and Disaster Medicine : The Official Journal of the National Association of EMS Physicians and the World Association for Emergency and Disaster Medicine in Association with the Acute Care Foundation* 25 (4): 289-295.

de Ville de Goyet, C. 2007. "Health Lessons Learned from the Recent Earthquakes and Tsunami in Asia." *Prehospital and Disaster Medicine: The Official Journal of the National Association of EMS Physicians and the World Association for Emergency and Disaster Medicine in Association with the Acute Care Foundation* 22 (1): 15-21.

de Ville de Goyet, C. 2008. "What Should We Learn from Recent Earthquakes in Asia?" *Prehospital and Disaster Medicine: The Official Journal of the National Association of EMS Physicians and the World Association for Emergency and Disaster Medicine in Association with the Acute Care Foundation* 23 (4): 305-307.

Dean, J.G., and H.J. Stain. 2010. "Mental Health Impact for Adolescents Living with Prolonged Drought." *The Australian Journal of Rural Health* 18 (1): 32-37.

Deebaj, R., M. Castren, and G. Ohlen. 2011. "Asia Tsunami Disaster 2004: Experience at Three International Airports." *Prehospital and Disaster Medicine: The Official Journal of the National Association of EMS Physicians and the World Association for Emergency and Disaster Medicine in Association with the Acute Care Foundation* 26 (1): 71-75.

Diaz, J.H. 2011. "The Legacy of the Gulf Oil Spill: Analyzing Acute Public Health Effects and Predicting Chronic Ones in Louisiana." *American Journal of Disaster Medicine* 6 (1): 5-22.

Dowell, S.F., J.W. Tappero, and T.R. Frieden. 2011. "Public Health in Haiti— Challeges and Progress." *New England Journal of Medicine* 364 (4): 300-301.

Du, W., G.J. FitzGerald, M. Clark, and X.Y. Hou. 2010. "Health Impacts of Floods." *Prehospital and Disaster Medicine: The Official Journal of the National Association of EMS Physicians and the World Association for Emergency and Disaster Medicine in association with the Acute Care Foundation* 25 (3): 265-272.

Ebi, K.L., M. Helmer, and J. Vainio. 2008. "The Health Impacts of Climate Change: Getting Started on a New Theme." *Prehospital and Disaster Medicine: The Official Journal of the National Association of EMS Physicians and the World Association for Emergency and Disaster Medicine in Association with the Acute Care Foundation* 23: s60-s64.

Englande, A.J., Jr. 2008. "Katrina and the Thai Tsunami—Water Quality and Public Health Aspects Mitigation and Research Needs." *International Journal of Environmental Research and Public Health* 5 (5): 384-393.

Friel, S., K. Bowen, D. Campbell-Lendrum, H. Frumkin, A.J. McMichael, and K. Rasanathan. 2011. "Climate Change, Noncommunicable Diseases, and Development: The Relationships and Common Policy Opportunities." *Annual Review of Public Health* 32: 133-147.

Gavilan, R.G., and J. Martinez-Urtaza. 2011. "[Environmental Drivers of Emergence and Spreading of Vibrio Epidemics in South America.]" *Revista Peruana de Medicina Experimental y Salud Publica* 28 (1): 109-115.

Guha-Sapir, D., and W.G. van Panhuis. 2009. "Health Impact of the 2004 Andaman Nicobar Earthquake and Tsunami in Indonesia." *Prehospital and Disaster Medicine: The Official Journal of the National Association of EMS Physicians and the World Association for Emergency and Disaster Medicine in Association with the Acute Care Foundation* 24 (6): 493-499.

Gupta, S.K., A. Suantio, A. Gray, E. Widyastuti, N. Jain, R. Rolos, R.M. Hoekstra, and R. Quick. 2007. "Factors Associated with E. coli Contamination of Household Drinking Water among Tsunami and Earthquake Survivors, Indonesia." *The American Journal of Tropical Medicine and Hygiene* 76 (6): 1158-1162.

Hashizume, M., A.S.G. Faruque, T. Terao, M.D. Yunus, K. Streatfield, T. Yamamoto, and K. Moji. 2011. "The Indian Ocean Dipole and Cholera Incidence in Bangladesh: A Time-series Analysis." *Environmental Health Perspectives* 119 (2): 239-244.

Horton, G., L. Hanna, and B. Kelly. 2010. "Drought, Drying and Climate Change: Emerging Health Issues for Ageing Australians in Rural Areas." *Australasian Journal on Ageing* 29 (1): 2-7.

Huq, A., M. Yunus, S.S. Sohel, A. Bhuiya, M. Emch, S.P. Luby, E. Russek-Cohen, G.B. Nair, R.B. Sack, and R.R. Colwell. 2010. "Simple Sari Cloth

Filtration of Water is Sustainable and Continues to Protect Villagers from Cholera in Matlab, Bangladesh." mBio 1 (1).

Ivers, L.C., P. Farmer, C.P. Almazor, and F. Leandre. 2010. "Five Complementary Interventions to Slow Cholera: Haiti." *Lancet* 376 (9758): 2048-2051.

Kalis, M.A., and R.J. Wilson. 2009. "Public Health and Drought." *Journal of Environmental Health* 72: 10-11.

Kanungo, R., Shashikala, I. Karunasagar, S. Srinivasan, D. Sheela, K. Venkatesh, and P. Anitha. 2007. "Contamination of Community Water Sources by Potentially Pathogenic Vibrios Following Sea Water Inundation." *The Journal of Communicable Diseases* 39 (4): 229-232.

Karmakar, S., A.S. Rathore, S.M. Kadri, S. Dutt, S. Khare, and S. Lal. 2008. "Post-earthquake Outbreak of Rotavirus Gastroenteritis in Kashmir (India): An Epidemiological Analysis." *Public Health* 122 (10): 981-989.

Keim, M.E. 2008. "Building Human Resilience: The Role of Public Health Preparedness and Response as an Adaptation to Climate Change." *American Journal of Preventive Medicine* 35 (5): 508-516.

Kistin, E.J., J. Fogarty, R.S. Pokrasso, M. McCally, and P.G. McCornick. 2010. "Climate Change, Water Resources and Child Health." *Archives of Disease in Childhood* 95 (7): 545-549.

Koelle, K. and D.A. Rasmussen. Influenza: prediction is worth a shot. (2014) *Nature.* 507 (7490), pp. 47-48

Llewellyn, M. 2006. "Floods and Tsunamis." *The Surgical Clinics of North America* 86 (3): 557-578.

Magan, M., K.M. Bile, B.M. Kazi, and Z. Gardezi. 2010. "Safe Water Supply in Emergencies and The Need for an Exit Strategy to Sustain Health Gains: Lessons Learned from the 2005 Earthquake in Pakistan." *Eastern Mediterranean Health Journal* 16 (Supplement): S91-S97.

Martinez-Urtaza, J., B. Huapaya, R.G. Gavilan, V. Blanco-Abad, J. Ansede-Bermejo, C. Cadarso-Suarez, A. Figueiras, and J. Trinanes. 2008. "Emergence of Asiatic Vibrio diseases in South America in phase with El Nino." *Epidemiology* 19 (6): 829-837.

Mason, V., H. Andrews, and D. Upton. 2010. "The Psychological Impact of Exposure to Floods." *Psychology, Health & Medicine* 15 (1): 61-73.

Math, S.B., J.P. John, S.C. Girimaji, V. Benegal, B. Sunny, K. Krishnakanth, U. Kumar, A. Hamza, S. Tandon, K. Jangam, K.S. Meena, B. Chandramukhi, and D. Nagaraja. 2008. "Comparative Study of Psychiatric Morbidity Among the Displaced and Non-Displaced Populations in the Andaman and Nicobar Islands Following the Tsunami." *Prehospital and Disaster Medicine: The Official Journal of the National Association of EMS Physicians and the World Association for Emergency and Disaster Medicine in Association with the Acute Care Foundation* 23 (1): 29-34; discussion 35.

Matsumoto, M., and K. Inoue. 2011. "Earthquake, Tsunami, Radiation Leak, and Crisis in Rural Health in Japan." *Rural and Remote Health* 11 (1): 1759.

McCann, D.G.C. 2009. "Preparing for the Worst." *The Journal of Legal Medicine* 30 (3): 329-348.

McCann, D.G.C. 2011. "A Review of Hurricane Disaster Planning for the Elderly." *World Medical and Health Policy* 3 (1): article 2.

McCann, D.G.C. and H.P. Cordi. 2011. "Developing International Standards for Disaster Preparedness and Response: How Do We Get There?" *World Medical and Health Policy* 3 (1): article 5.

McCauley, L.A. 2010. "Environments and Health: Will the BP Oil Spill Affect Our Health?" *The American Journal of Nursing* 110 (9): 54-56.

McLaughlin, K.A., J.A. Fairbank, M.J. Gruber, R.T. Jones, J.D. Osofsky, B. Pfefferbaum, N.A. Sampson, and R.C. Kessler. 2010. "Trends in Serious Emotional Disturbance Among Youths Exposed to Hurricane Katrina." *Journal of the American Academy of Child and Adolescent Psychiatry* 49 (10): 990-1000, 1000 e1-2.

Meo, S.A., A.M. Al-Drees, S. Rasheed, I.M. Meo, M.M. Al-Saadi, H.A. Ghani, and J.R. Alkandari. 2009. "Health Complaints Among Subjects Involved in Oil Cleanup Operations During Oil Spillage from a Greek Tanker "Tasman Spirit"." *International Journal of Occupational Medicine and Environmental Health* 22 (2): 143-148.

Morrow, R.C., and D.M. Llewellyn. 2006. "Tsunami Overview." *Military Medicine* 171 (10 Suppl 1): 5-7.

Murthy, S., and M.D. Christian. 2010. "Infectious Diseases Following Disasters." *Disaster*

Medicine and Public Health Preparedness 4 (3): 232-238.

Nahar, P., F. Alamgir, A.E. Collins, and A. Bhuiya. 2010. "Contextualizing Disaster in Relation to Human Health in Bangladesh." *Asian Journal of Water, Environment and Pollution* 7 (1): 55-62.

Nicogossian, A., T. Zimmerman, O. Kloiber, A. Grigoriev, N. Koizumi, J. Heineman-Pieper, J.D. Mayer, C.R. Doarn, and W. Jacobs. 2011. "Disaster Medicine: The Need for Global Action." *World Medical and Health Policy* 3 (1): Article 1.

Normile, D. 2011. "Japan Disaster." Waves of Destruction. *Science* 331 (6023): 1376.

Ohtomo, K., N. Kobayashi, A. Sumi, and N. Ohtomo. 2010. "Relationship of Cholera Incidence to El Nino and Solar Activity Elucidated by Time-series Analysis. *Epidemiology and Infection* 138 (1): 99-107.

Okumura, J., T. Kai, Z. Hayati, F. Karmil, K. Kimura, and Y. Yamamoto. 2009. "Antimicrobial Therapy for Water-Associated Wound Infections in a Disaster Setting: Gram-negative Bacilli in an Aquatic Environment and Lessons from Banda Aceh." *Prehospital and Disaster Medicine: The Official Journal of the National Association of EMS Physicians and the World Association for Emergency and Disaster Medicine in Association with the Acute Care Foundation* 24 (3): 189-196.

Olago, D., M. Marshall, S.O. Wandiga, M. Opondo, P.Z. Yanda, R. Kanalawe, A.K. Githeko, T. Downs, A. Opere, R. Kavumvuli, E. Kirumira, L. Ogallo, P. Mugambi, E. Apindi, F. Githui, J. Kathuri, L. Olaka, R. Sigalla, R. Nanyunja, T. Baguma, and P. Achola. 2007. "Climatic, Socio-economic, and Health Factors Affecting Human Vulnerability to Cholera in the Lake Victoria Basin, East Africa." *Ambio* 36 (4): 350-358.

Olteanu, A., R. Arnberger, R. Grant, C. Davis, D. Abramson, and J. Asola. 2011. "Persistence of Mental Health Needs Among Children Affected by Hurricane Katrina in New Orleans." *Prehospital and Disaster Medicine: The Official Journal of the National Association of EMS Physicians and the World Association for Emergency and Disaster Medicine in Association with the Acute Care Foundation* 26 (1): 3-6.

Paul, S.K., and J.K. Routray. 2010. "Flood Proneness and Coping Strategies: The Experiences of Two Villages in Bangladesh." *Disasters* 34 (2): 489-508.

Peek, L., and L.M. Stough. 2010. "Children with Disabilities in the Context of Disaster: A Social Vulnerability Perspective." *Child Development* 81 (4): 1260-1270.

Prasartritha, T., R. Tungsiripat, and P. Warachit. 2008. "The Revisit of 2004 Tsunami in Thailand: Characteristics of Wounds." *International Wound Journal* 5 (1): 8-19.

Rahardjo, E., K. Wiroatmodjo, and P. Koeshartono. 2008. "Toward More Efficient Multinational Work on Rescue and Aid for Disasters: Lessons Learned During the Aceh Tsunami and Yogya Earthquake." *Prehospital and Disaster Medicine : The Official Journal of the National Association of EMS Physicians and the World Association for Emergency and Disaster Medicine in Association with the Acute Care Foundation* 23 (4): 301-304.

Raphael, B., M. Taylor, G. Stevens, M. Barr, M. Gorringe, and K. Agho. 2009. "Factors Associated with Population Risk Perceptions of Continuing Drought in Australia." *The Australian Journal of Rural Health* 17 (6): 330-337.

Red Cross. 2009.
http://www.redcross.org/www-files/Documents/pdf/Preparedness/checklists/Flood.pdf (accessed April 5, 2011).

Sabucedo, J.M., C. Arce, C. Senra, G. Seoane, and I. Vazquez. 2010. "Symptomatic Profile and Health-Related Quality of Life of Persons Affected by the Prestige Catastrophe." *Disasters* 34 (3): 809-820.

Saniotis, A., and P. Bi. 2009. "Global Warming and Australian Public Health: Reasons to be Concerned." *Australian Health Review: A Publication of the Australian Hospital Association* 33 (4): 611-617.

Shimi, A.C., G.A. Parvin, C. Biswas, and R. Shaw. 2010. "Impact and Adaptation to Flood: A Focus on Water Supply, Sanitation and Health Problems of Rural Community in Bangladesh." *Disaster Prevention and Management* 19 (3): 298-313.

Taye, A., D.H. Mariam, and V. Murray. 2010. "Interim Report: Review of Evidence of the Health Impact of Famine in Ethiopia." *Perspectives in Public Health* 130 (5): 222-226.

United Nations Office for the Coordination of Human Affairs (UN OCHA). 2011. http://www.unocha.org/top-stories/all-stories/japan-recovery-operation-missing-persons-tsunami-aftermath-0 (accessed April 28, 2011).

von Schreeb, J., L. Riddez, H. Samnegard, and H. Rosling. 2008. "Foreign Field Hospitals in the Recent Sudden-Onset Disasters in Iran, Haiti, Indonesia, and Pakistan." *Prehospital and Disaster Medicine: The Official*

Journal of the National Association of EMS Physicians and the World Association for Emergency and Disaster Medicine in association with the Acute Care Foundation 23 (2): 144-151; discussion 152-153.

Wahlquist, A.K. 2009. "Water and Its Role in Food and Health Security--the Importance of Water to Food Production." *Asia Pacific Journal of Clinical Nutrition* 18 (4): 501-506.

Walton, D.A., and L.C. Ivers. 2011. "Responding to Cholera in Post-Earthquake Haiti." *The New England Journal of Medicine* 364 (1): 3-5.

Wang, G., R.B. Minnis, J.L. Belant, and C.L. Wax. 2010. "Dry Weather Induces Outbreaks of Human West Nile Virus Infections." *BMC Infectious Diseases* 10: 38.

WHO. 1998. *Health Sector Emergency Preparedness Guide.* Geneva: WHO.

WHO. 2010. "Water and Sanitation in Health Emergencies: The Role of WHO in the Response to the Earthquake in Haiti, 12 January 2010." Releve Epidemiologique Hebdomadaire/Section d'hygiene du Secretariat de la Societe des Nations = Weekly Epidemiological Record/Health Section of the Secretariat of the League of Nations 85 (36): 349-354.

Zhang, J., D.L. Mauzerall, T. Zhu, S. Liang, M. Ezzati, and J.V. Remais. 2010. "Environmental Health in China: Progress Towards Clean Air and Safe Water." *Lancet* 375 (9720): 1110-1119.

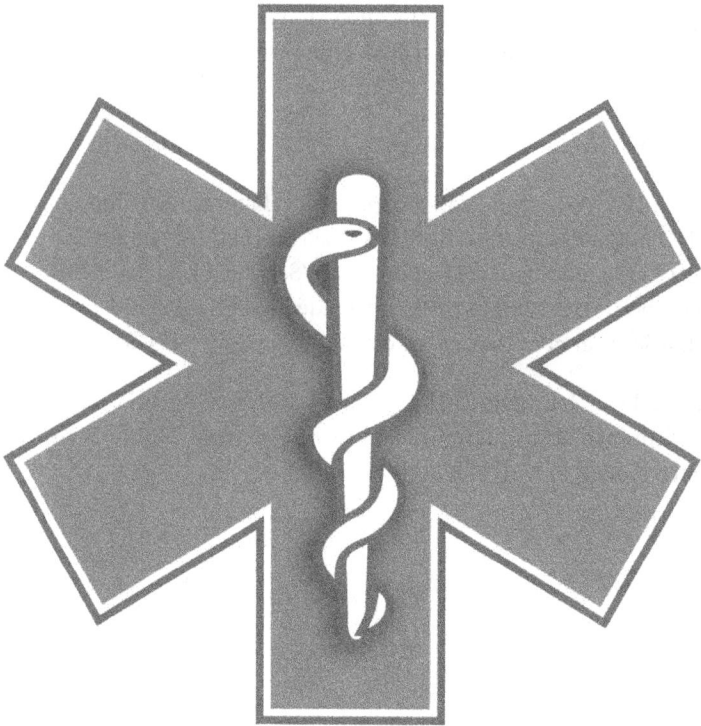

CYBER SECURITY THREATS TO PUBLIC HEALTH

Daniel J. Barnett, *Johns Hopkins Bloomberg School of Public Health*
Tara Kirk Sell, *Johns Hopkins Bloomberg School of Public Health*
Robert K. Lord, *Johns Hopkins University School of Medicine*
Curtis J. Jenkins, *U.S. Navy Information Dominance Corps Reserve Command*
James W. Terbush, *Science and Technology Directorate, NORAD*
Thomas A. Burke, *Johns Hopkins Bloomberg School of Public Health*

INTRODUCTION

The vulnerability of the public's health to cybersecurity threats has received insufficient attention in the research literature to date and has yet to be well understood (Harries and Yellowlees 2012). This paper is intended as a step toward analyzing cyber-related public health challenges in a systematic fashion. The research gaps on cybersecurity and public health are particularly striking in light of an April 2012 report by the Government Accountability Office, which noted not only the ever-increasing prevalence of cybersecurity threats ("cyber threats"), but also the many intentional and unintentional sources from which such threats can originate, the numerous targets that malicious actors might exploit, and the varied tools at the disposal of those who would seek to launch cyber attacks (U.S. Government Accountability Office 2012a). The adage noted by security expert Bruce Schneier in his 2012 Science piece rings truer with each passing day: "Everything gets hacked (Schneier 2012)."

With the increased funding for health information technology through such legislation as the Health Information Technology for Economic and Clinical Health (HITECH) Act (Centers for Disease Control and Prevention

2012) comes an increased need to protect health information and public health infrastructure (Hathaway 2009; Editorial 2009). Indeed, the healthcare sector has been described in the literature as a "tantalizing opportunity" for cyberterrorism (Harries and Yellowlees 2012). However, as noted in 2011, the focus in peer-reviewed literature has been more on the role of information technology during emergencies and less on how electronic systems would respond to threats themselves (McGowan, Cusack, and Bloomrosen 2011). The U.S. government reports provide perhaps the richest cyber threat response literature, but even here details regarding the specific effects of cyber threats on public health and strategies for threat mitigation is lacking. Healthcare seems to "[lag] behind the other critical industries, mostly because of its diverse, fragmented nature and a relative lack of regulation when compared with, say, the energy industry (Colias 2004)." In this paper, we briefly describe the effect of cyber threats on several aspects of public health and suggest future research to better characterize this problem and determine policy solutions.

CYBERSECURITY AND THE PUBLIC HEALTH EMERGENCY PREPAREDNESS SYSTEM

In 2008, the Institute of Medicine presented a seven-stakeholders framework for the Public Health Emergency Preparedness System, comprising (1) HealthCare Delivery System, (2) Homeland Security and Public Safety, (3) Employers and Businesses, (4) The Media, (5) Academia, (6) Communities, and (7) Governmental Public Health Infrastructure, the last of which serves as an organizational hub for the other participants (Altevogt et al. 2008). This framework (Figure 1) offers a useful analytic lens for understanding the interconnected elements collectively essential for public health emergency readiness—and by extension, provides a window into how these vital elements may be critically endangered by cyber threats. While the framework does not explicitly mention information technology, such technology is nonetheless heavily utilized by (and represents a potential significant security vulnerability for) each of its seven stakeholders, and thus infuses all elements of this system.

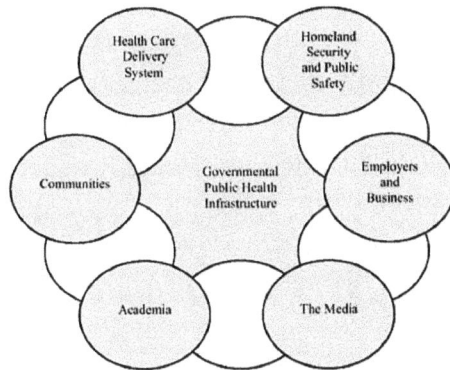

Figure 1. The Public Health Emergency Preparedness System (Institute of Medicine [2008] as adapted from the Institute of Medicine, *The Future of the Public's Health in the 21st Century* [2002])

Of relevance here, cyber threats to these seven-stakeholder elements can be classified in terms of their capacity to effect (1) Losses of Integrity, (2) Losses of Availability, (3) Losses of Confidentiality and (4) Physical Destruction in systems that contribute to public health (U.S. Army Training and Doctrine Command 2005). We note parenthetically which of these categories apply to the threats described below.

HEALTHCARE DELIVERY SYSTEM

The HealthCare Delivery System represents the front-line healthcare providers in the United States, such as hospitals and emergency medical services providers. The effects of power outages on hospitals caused by the collapse of public power grids (U.S. Government Accountability Office 2012b) or the destruction of generators due to modifying code in Programmable Logic Controllers would have devastating consequences for patient care (Physical Destruction) (Choo 2011). There are also more subtle threats such as the theft or loss of patient information (Confidentiality) (Martin 2001), disruption of care due to software outages (Availability) (Lichtenfels 2012), or loss of confidence in healthcare providers due to perceptions of inadequate security (Integrity) (McGowan, Cusack, and Bloomrosen 2011), the latter of which could decrease utilization of needed services. A newly emergent threat is the potential for security and privacy risks that emerge in personal medical devices, given their increasingly networked and wireless nature (Confidentiality/Physical Destruction) (Kramer et al. 2012; Avancha, Baxi, and Kotz 2013).

HOMELAND SECURITY AND PUBLIC SAFETY

Homeland Security and Public Safety actors could be affected by a wide array of cyber threats, such as disruption of emergency telephone lines and EMS systems, which could slow or disable emergency medical response (Availability/Integrity) (Kun 2002). The role of Homeland Security and Public Safety is also important in managing threats that combine cyber elements with more traditional weaponry. In 2002, the Director of the National Infrastructure Protection Center stated that his greatest fear was "a physical attack in conjunction with a successful cyber-attack," a situation that could amplify the public health impact of weapons of mass destruction (WMDs) or conventional weapons (Gellman 2002). However, while the Department of Homeland Security (DHS) has elevated the importance of cybersecurity, it still faces challenges coordinating and effecting change in this area (Lord and Sharp 2011).

EMPLOYERS AND BUSINESSES

Traditional cyber threats to businesses present a range of damages that include reputational damage, financial gain and fraud, commercial advantage and/or economic and political damage (Confidentiality /Integrity) (Scully 2011). Any and all of these activities could disrupt the providing of public health resources through an inability to produce needed medical equipment or drugs through manufacturing stoppages (Availability) (De Oliveira, Theilken, and McCarthy 2011), loss of protected health information and subsequent decreases in public trust of health apparatuses (Loss of Integrity) (McGowan, Cusack, and Bloomrosen 2011) or failures of vendors to provide key hospital services that might range from software to temporary staffing (Availability). In addition, since the Aurora Test in 2007, and the Stuxnet virus of 2010, it has been clear that the potential for users to remotely access and damage physical systems is all-too-real (U.S. Government Accountability Office 2012b), and dangerous when applied to the many functions performed by businesses, particularly regulated utilities (Physical Destruction). The above-noted threats, if they occurred in businesses critical to public health infrastructure, could shut down or slow supply chains, impair patient care, and impede emergency response, potentially leading to significant loss of life.

THE MEDIA

The media serve to transmit "legitimated" information as provided by government and expert sources (Wray et al. 2004), and to the extent that cyber threats have the potential to corrupt or distort this information, they can detract from the ability of these critical structures to aid in public health (Integrity). Even more simply, cyber threats that directly or indirectly disable media transmission or reception impair the ability of actors in this model to reach communities with up-to-date information (Availability). There also exists the potential for social media to contribute to public health response (U.S. Department of Homeland Security 2012), and to the extent that this capability is utilized, it may present a corresponding vulnerability (Integrity/Availability).

COMMUNITIES

Communities are highly vulnerable to the public health effects of the failure of cyber-based systems, as they often lack the backup generators and systems that government or industry actors might have. Food and medication may lose their refrigeration, and medical apparatuses outside of hospitals may be vulnerable to power loss (Physical Destruction/Availability) (Clem, Galwankar, and Buck 2003). Social discontent and unrest are potential consequences of community disruption, with obvious public health consequences if such unrest is large scale and prolonged in nature (Choo 2011).

ACADEMIA

While academia may not play a core role during a cyber threat beyond providing expert advice (Wray et al. 2004), it plays a critical role in preparation for such threats (Institute of Medicine 2002). One exception to these primarily preparative and advisory roles, however, is the threat of sensitive academic research with uses that could either be weaponizable or induce some manner of public health crisis (Confidentiality) (Schneier 2012). In this case, cyber threats could pose very real dangers, by arming malicious actors with decidedly non-virtual armaments. Moreover, academic campuses are vulnerable to power outages due to cyber threats, given that their laboratories house infectious agents, cadavers, and a host of research animals (Physical Destruction).

GOVERNMENTAL PUBLIC HEALTH INFRASTRUCTURE

Our final actor, Government Public Health Infrastructure, has many roles that could be disrupted by cyber threats. Such initiatives as the CDC's Select Agent Program (Lister 2005) could be subject to cyber threats that penetrate and improperly release information that could cause or exacerbate public health crises, given that this work focuses on dangerous agents and potential countermeasures (Confidentiality). Some components of the public health supply chain could be rendered unusable by cyber threats, such as elements of the Strategic National Stockpile (Lister 2005) that require refrigeration or electricity (Physical Destruction). Finally, the availability of command and control infrastructure could be impaired during cyberattacks, limiting HHS's ability to coordinate public health response and conduct surveillance on the progress of efforts (Availability/

Integrity). Indeed, the critical analytical role of health informaticians in public health surveillance and analysis (Centers for Disease Control and Prevention 2012) could be disrupted through threats to data collection, storage, and analysis similar to those faced by businesses.

In the context of the seven-actor framework discussed above (Altevogt et al 2008), we note that perhaps the most vulnerable components, significantly exposed to all four types of cyber threats, are those of the HealthCare Delivery System, Businesses and Employers, and the Governmental Public Health Infrastructure. Indirectly, long-term burdens on communities due to cyber-threats that disable communication and public utilities can tax the other public health actors such that their best efforts could be insufficient in controlling community discontent. While disruptions to media and academia may be less overtly deleterious to public health, they nonetheless pose serious risks as noted above. Thus, disruptions in any of the seven actors due to cyber threats have potentially serious consequences for public health, though these consequences are currently ill-defined due to a dearth of peer-reviewed literature in this area.

CYBERSECURITY AND ESSENTIAL PUBLIC HEALTH SERVICES: A CROSSWALK ANALYSIS

A crosswalk analysis of the potential impacts of cyber threats on essential public health services further highlights the extensive implications of cybersecurity for population health and wellbeing (Figure 2). The CDC-defined 10 essential public health services include: (1) monitor health status to identify and solve community health problems; (2) diagnose and investigate health problems and health hazards in the community; (3) inform, educate, and empower people about health issues; (4) mobilize community partnerships and action to identify and solve health problems; (5) develop policies and plans that support individual and community health efforts; (6) enforce laws and regulations that protect health and ensure safety; (7) link people to needed personal health services and assure the provision of healthcare when otherwise unavailable; (8) assure competent public and personal healthcare work-force; (9) evaluate effectiveness, accessibility, and quality of personal and population-based health services; and 10) research for new insights and innovative solutions to health problems (Centers for Disease Control and Prevention 2010).

Figure 2. Ten Essential Public Health Services and Cyber Threats Crosswalk

1. MONITOR health status to identify and solve community health problems

- Key activity affected: Health surveillance

   Computer systems that collect, transfer and store data are vital for both active and passive surveillance. Loss of these systems through direct attack or loss of infrastructure would limit the ability of PH to track and monitor diseases and health conditions of importance.

2. DIAGNOSE AND INVESTIGATE health problems and health hazards in the community

- Key activity affected: Analysis of health information

   Loss of access to information hinders the ability of health departments to diagnose problems in the community. While health investigations may continue, loss of infrastructure, such as communications channels could prevent timely analysis of health problems and access to laboratory and hospital data.

3. INFORM, EDUCATE, and empower people about health issues

- Key activity affected: Delivery of health information

   Attack on public health information dissemination systems could limit the ability of the health department to disseminate information. Loss of infrastructure could prevent people from receiving important information.

4. MOBILIZE community partnerships and action to identify and solve health problems

- Activities in this area may provide resilience in the face of cyber threats

    Coalitions, partnerships, and motivated stakeholders may be able to continue communication and activity through relationships formed before disaster. These activities may help communities weather the loss of infrastructure or provide alternate conduits of information flow. However, the loss of electronic communication could reduce the effectiveness of coalitions such as hospital coalitions when they are needed the most.

5. DEVELOP POLICIES AND PLANS that support individual and community health efforts

- Activities in this area may improve both prevention and response in the face of cyber threats

    Educating policymakers on the public health effects of cyber threats to formulate better policy and planning for possible response activities before disaster could reduce the effects of cyber threats.

6. ENFORCE laws and regulations that protect health and ensure safety

- Activities in this area could help to reduce the impact of cyber threats

    Encouraging hospitals and other relevant organizations to improve practices and reduce vulnerabilities could reduce impacts of cyber threats. However, the loss of infrastructure could reduce the ability to communicate notifiable diseases or health violations.

7. LINK people to needed personal health services and assure the provision of healthcare when otherwise unavailable

- Key activity affected: Increased need to respond to public health emergencies in order to provide people with necessary health services

Loss of infrastructure would cause the denial of utility services needed to maintain the health of the public. Loss of electricity or water during heat waves or cold spells will require response from public health to prevent loss of life. Similarly, cyber attacks may result in the failures of industrial safety systems (e.g. in chemical manufacturing) that could cause widespread illness and possibly death, requiring response from public health entities.

- Key activity affected: Loss of access to appropriate medical care

  Hospitals may encounter reduced capacity to provide medical care through the loss of hospital systems. Additionally, loss of access to health records limit public health's ability to provide appropriate care, shelter, and medicine in times of need. Damage to infrastructure such as transit or insurance/payment methods could also prevent people from accessing necessary medical care.

8. ASSURE competent public and personal healthcare workforce

- Creeping losses in this health service will exacerbate problems posed by Cyber threats

  The continuing loss of staff and funding make it difficult for health departments to meet community needs for public and personal health services. Increased strain on the system due to cyber threats will only magnify this problem. Additionally, cyber threats may reduce workers' ability to access just-in-time training.

9. EVALUATE effectiveness, accessibility, and quality of personal and population-based health services

- Key activity affected: Assessment of public health interventions

  Evaluation of health interventions requires data storage and communication to measure progress toward goals. In an information or communication poor environment it may be difficult to know if the work public health is doing is making a difference.

10. RESEARCH for new insights and innovative solutions to health problems

- Activities in this area will help identify gaps, harden public health systems, and build coping strategies for vulnerabilities that cannot be addressed. However, research during a cyber crisis may be limited due to loss of infrastructure and records.

As Figure 2 illustrates, virtually every essential service of public health may face significant operational impacts from cybersecurity vulnerabilities. While a more granular discussion of the numerous specific activities impacted within each essential service is beyond the scope of discussion here and insufficiently addressed by the peer-reviewed literature to date, this paper nonetheless reveals critical challenges that cybersecurity poses to both routine and emergent public health activities and systems.

DISCUSSION

In this paper we have taken initial steps to examine intersections between cybersecurity and public health, through the lenses of the public health emergency preparedness system and the essential services of public health. Given the paucity of rigorous research to date on this nascent public health threat, any formal policy recommendations would be premature. However, our preliminary analyses described above permit at least a broad-based discussion of vital policy and research considerations moving forward, which we describe below.

IMPROVED PRIVATE–PUBLIC PARTNERSHIP

As we have noted, the public health emergency preparedness system comprises an array of different stakeholders. It should come as no surprise that increasing the resilience of the public health system to cyber-attack will require partnership between the private sector and government (Centers for Disease Control and Prevention 2012). Improved information sharing between different entities is an important step toward creating a unified set of objectives pertaining to cybersecurity. Additionally, members of the healthcare delivery system, homeland security and public safety, employers and businesses, the media, communities and academia should work with public health to ensure that any government policy in cybersecurity takes into account the broad set of interests that make up the public health emergency preparedness system. Finally, the innovative capacity of the private sector should be leveraged to address cybersecurity concerns (Lord and Sharp 2011).

RECOGNITION OF PUBLIC HEALTH ASPECT OF CYBERSECURITY BY POLICYMAKERS

It is clear that a cyber-attack could have far-reaching consequences on the nation's economy, intellectual property, sensitive military information, and critical infrastructure. Here, we add another dimension—the health of the public. Recently, the Secretary of Defense, Leon Panetta stated, "The collective result of these kinds of attacks could be a cyber Pearl Harbor; an attack that would cause physical destruction and the loss of life (Panetta 2012)." Our analysis supports this premise, highlighting how cyber-attacks may critically endanger vital public health elements, possibly resulting in serious health consequences. Policymakers should understand the consequences of a lack of preparedness for cyber-attacks. Future legislation and regulations in this space should also account for the interactions between cybersecurity and public health.

FUTURE RESEARCH AVENUES

Ultimately, significant new research is required to more thoroughly understand the complex risk relationships between cybersecurity and public health and to develop rigorous evidence-based policy and practices to address this multifaceted public health threat. Such efforts will necessarily entail identifying public health indicators of relevance to cybersecurity threats; assessing public health system functioning based on these indicators (and potentially new indicators as they arise); providing health practitioners, policymakers, and researchers with timely access to these indicators; and facilitating cybersecurity-related public health risk communication activities for these respective stakeholder audiences. Additionally, interdisciplinary research collaborations will be essential to bringing stakeholders with vastly different experience together around this multidimensional public health threat.

REFERENCES

Altevogt, B.M., et al., eds. 2008. "Institute of Medicine." *Research Priorities in Emergency Preparedness and Response for Public Health Systems: A Letter Report*. Washington, D.C.: The National Academies Press. http://books.nap.edu/openbook.php?record_id=12136&page=12 (accessed August 1, 2012).

Anonymous. 2009. "Wanted: Cyber-czars [editorial]." *Nature* 458 (7241): 945.

Avancha, S., A. Baxi, and D. Kotz. 2013 [accepted, in press]. "Privacy in Mobile Technology for Personal Healthcare." ACM Computing Surveys 45 (1). Pre-print: http://www.cs.dartmouth.edu/~dfk/papers/avancha-survey.pdf (accessed August 5, 2012).

Centers for Disease Control and Prevention. 2010. "National Public Health Performance Standards Program. 10 Essential Public Health Services." http://www.cdc.gov/nphpsp/essentialservices.html (accessed September 21, 2012).

Centers for Disease Control and Prevention. 2012. "CDC's Vision for Public Health Surveillance in the 21st Century." http://www.cdc.gov/mmwr/pdf/other/su6103.pdf (accessed August 1, 2012).

Choo, K.R. 2011. "The Cyber Threat Landscape: Challenges and Future Research Directions." *Computers and Security* 30: 719-731.

Clem, A., S. Galwankar, and G. Buck. 2003. "Health Implications of Cyber-Terrorism." *Prehospital and Disaster Medicine* 18 (3): 272-275.

Colias, M. 2004. "Cyber Security." *Hospitals and Health Networks*. http://www.hhnmag.com/hhnmag/jsp/articledisplay.

jsp?dcrpath=HHNMAG/PubsNewsArticle/data/backup/0405HHN_FEA_
Cyber_Security&domain=HHNMAG/ (accessed August 1, 2012).

De Oliveira, Jr. G.S., L.S. Theilken, and R.J. McCarthy. 2011. "Shortage of
Perioperative Drugs: Implications for Anesthesia Practice and Patient
Safety." *Anesthesia and Analgesia* 113 (6): 1429-1435.

Gellman, B. 2002. "Cyber Attacks by Al Qaeda Feared." Washington Post.
http://www.washingtonpost.com/wp-dyn/content/article/2006/06/12/
AR2006061200711.html (accessed August 5, 2012).

Harries, D., and P.M. Yellowlees. 2012. "Cyberterrorism: Is the U.S. Healthcare
System Safe?" *Telemedicine Journal of E Health* [Epub ahead of print].

Hathaway, M. 2009. "The President's Cyberspace Policy Review."
http://www.whitehouse.gov/CyberReview/ (accessed August 1, 2012).

Institute of Medicine. 2002. *The Future of the Public's Health in the 21st
Century*. Washington, DC: The National Academies Press.
http://iom.edu/Reports/2002/The-Future-of-the-Publics-Health-in-the-
21st-Century.aspx (accessed August 1, 2012).

Kramer, D.B., et al., 2012. "Security and Privacy Qualities of Medical Devices:
An Analysis of FDA Postmarket Surveillance." *PLoS One* 7 (7): 1-7.
http://www.plosone.org/article/info%3Adoi%2F10.1371%2Fjournal.
pone.0040200 (accessed August 6, 2012).

Kun, L.G. 2002. "Homeland Security: The Possible, Probable, and Perils of
Information Technology. Information Technology Is a Key Component in
Both Defending Against and Aiding Terrorism Threats." *IEEE Engineering
in Medicine and Biology* 21 (5): 28-33.

Lichtenfels, R. 2012. US Department of Homeland Security. "US Department
of Homeland Security's Cybersecurity and Communications Integration
Center." Presented at Spring Conference of Information Systems Audit and
Control Association; April 30, 2012; New York, NY.
http://www.isaca.org/chapters2/New-York-Metropolitan/membership/
Documents/2012-04-30%20Spring%20Conference-Meeting/2%20
Lichtenfels%20DHS%20NCCIC%202.pdf (accessed August 2, 2012).

Lister, S.A. 2005. Congressional Research Service. An Overview of the U.S.
Public Health System in the Context of Emergency Preparedness.
http://www.fas.org/sgp/crs/homesec/RL31719.pdf (accessed August 3, 2012).

Lord, K.M., and T. Sharp, eds. 2011. Center for a New American Security. *America's Cyber Future: Security and Prosperity in the Information Age*: Volume 1. http://www.cnas.org/files/documents/publications/CNAS_Cyber_Volume%20I_0.pdf (accessed August 4, 2012).

Martin, R.A. 2001. "Managing Vulnerabilities in Networked Systems." *Computer* 34 (11): 32-38.

McGowan, J.J., C.M. Cusack, and M. Bloomrosen. 2011. "The Future of Health IT Innovation and Informatics: A Report from AMIA's 2010 Policy Meeting." *Journal of the American Medical Informatics Association: JAMIA* 19: 460-467.

Panetta, Leon E. U.S. Department of Defense. "Remarks by Secretary Panetta on Cybersecurity to the Business Executives for National Security." Presented in New York City, on October 11, 2012. http://www.defense.gov/transcripts/transcript.aspx?transcriptid=5136 (accessed November 28, 2012).

Schneier, B. 2012. "Securing Medical Research: A Cybersecurity Point of View." *Science* 336 (6088): 1527-1529.

Scully, T. 2011. "The Cyber Threat, Trophy Information and the Fortress Mentality." *J Business Continuity & Emergency Planning* 5 (3): 195-207. http://www.ncbi.nlm.nih.gov/pubmed/22130338 (accessed August 1, 2012).

U.S. Army Training and Doctrine Command. 2005. Cyber Operations and Cyber Terrorism. *DCSINT Handbook* No. 1.02. http://www.dtic.mil/cgi-bin/GetTRDoc?Location=U2&doc=GetTRDoc.pdf&AD=ADA439217/ (accessed August 4, 2012).

U.S. Department of Homeland Security. 2012. *National Preparedness Report.* http://www.fema.gov/library/viewRecord.do?id=5914 (accessed August 3, 2012).

U.S. Government Accountability Office. 2012a. "Cybersecurity: Threats Impacting the Nation." http://www.gao.gov/products/GAO-12-666T (accessed August 1, 2012).

U.S. Government Accountability Office. 2012b. "Cybersecurity: Challenges in Securing the Electricity Grid." GAO-12-926T. http://www.gao.gov/products/GAO-12-926T (accessed August 1, 2012).

Wray R.J., et al. 2004. "Theoretical Perspectives on Public Communication Preparedness for Terrorist Attacks." *Family & Community Health* 27 (3): 232-241.

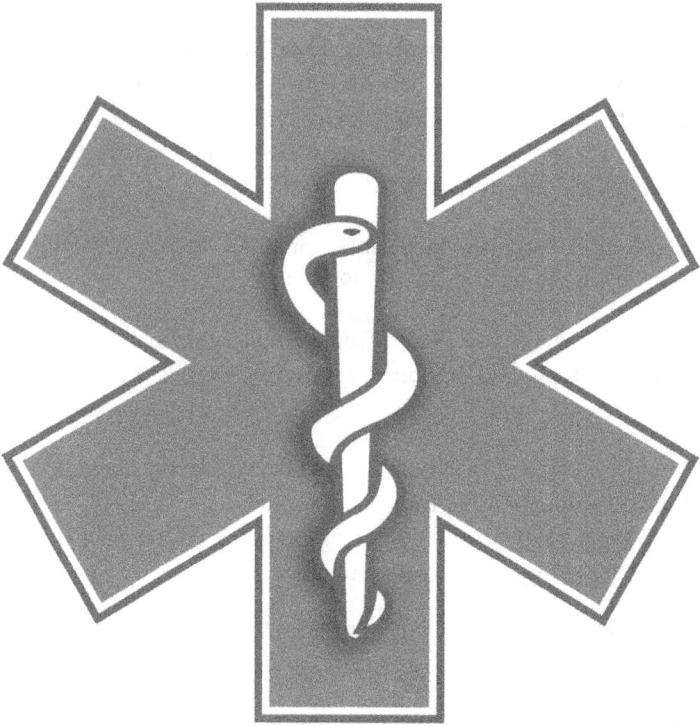

ANTI-MICROBIAL DRUG RESISTANCE: A HUMAN DISASTER IN THE MAKING

Arnauld Nicogossian, *George Mason Univeristy*
Thomas Zimmerman, *International Society of Microbial Resistance*
Otmar Kloiber, *World Medical Association*
Edward J. Septimus, *Texas A&M University*

According to the U.S. Centers for Disease Control and Prevention (CDC), the number of antibiotic-resistant pathogens is on the rise, creating a major public health problem and threatening advances in life-saving technologies, such as organ transplants, cancer therapy, and complex surgical procedures. Anti-microbial drug resistance (AMDR) is the ability of a specific microorganism to withstand a drug or a biocide preparation that interferes with its growth and functions (Meyers 1987; Russell 1997). Resistance usually involves gradation, rather than being an "all or none" phenomenon. Resistance and virulence are not related: a resistant pathogen may be no more virulent than an antibiotic-sensitive microorganism (Holmberg, Solomon, and Blake 1987). Resistance is a complex phenomenon involving the microorganism, the drug, the environment, and the patient, individually and in their complex interaction.

Bacteria have evolved protective mechanisms, primarily plasmids, to cope with and survive in the ever-changing environment (Russell 1997). Antibiotics, naturally produced by bacteria, existed long before humans discovered their properties and used them on an unprecedented scale. Bacteria had ample time to respond to harmful substances, develop and share defense mechanisms, and ensure their own survival. Humans coexist with many microorganisms, of which only a small subset presents a threat to health.

The 2008 global antibiotic market was estimated at USD24 billion and is projected to reach USD40.3 billion by 2015 (PRWeb 2011). Antibiotic drugs, including anti-viral, anti-helminthes, and anti-fungal preparations, are sold both for therapeutic and industrial (agricultural) uses. The agricultural consumption exceeds the therapeutic uses for this class of drugs. The rate of antibiotic prescriptions is on the rise in Greece, Croatia, Denmark, and Ireland both for out- and in-patient services. A modest downward trend (1998–2005) was reported for Belgium, the Czech Republic, France, Slovakia, Slovenia, Sweden, and the United Kingdom (Eurosurveillance 2008; Meropol, Chen, and Metlay 2009). In the United States and Japan, the overall antibiotic drugs usage remains high (Higashi and Furuhara 2009). Reliable estimates of global mortality and morbidity attributable to AMDR are lacking. Some experts are concerned that we are entering a dangerous "post antibiotic era" of a decreasing pipeline of new and effective antibiotics and rising trends in mortality from AMDR (Alanis 2005). The importance of AMDR threats has been recently highlighted by the World Health Organization (WHO 2011):

- Infections caused by resistant microorganisms often fail to respond to conventional treatment, resulting in prolonged illness and greater risk of death.

- About 440,000 new cases of multi-drug-resistant tuberculosis (MDR-TB) emerge annually, causing at least 150,000 deaths.

- Resistance to an earlier generation of anti-malarial preparations such as chloroquine and sulfadoxine-pyrimethamine is widespread in most malaria-endemic countries.

- A high percentage of hospital-acquired infections are caused by highly resistant bacteria such as methicillin-resistant Staphylococcus aureus (MRSA).

- Inappropriate and irrational use of anti-microbial drugs does provide a fertile environment for resistant microorganisms to emerge, spread, and persist.

It has been estimated that the economic burden of AMDR exceeds USD38 billion (Tucker 2010). Almost seven out of every 1,000 hospitalized patients (in developed economy countries) are either infected or carry microorganisms resistant to common antibiotic drugs. In U.S. hospitals, 96,000 patients contract nosocomial infection(s) annually. Nosocomial infections are among the 10 leading causes of death, claiming between 16,000 and 19,000 lives annually in the United States. The 2000 estimates by the European Union (EU) Hospitals (Kaier et al. 2008) showed that:

- 30–40% of cases are linked to cross-infection by the hands of healthcare workers (HCWs);

- 20–25% of cases are due to selective anti-microbial pressure;

- 20–25% of patients suffer from the introduction of new pathogens; and

- the remaining 20% of nosocomial infections result from the lack of proper control and oversight of antibiotic prescriptions (Weinstein 2001; Woodward et al. 1987).

Inappropriate use of antibiotic drugs is a major contributing factor to the spread of the AMDR pandemic. WHO reported that in 2005 more than 50% of all medicines (including antibiotic drugs) were prescribed, dispensed, or sold inappropriately, with at least 50% of all patients failing to take them correctly (WHO 2010). Countries which implemented policies on the appropriate usage of antibiotics had a positive effect on AMDR (Awad, Ball, and Eltayeb 2007; Isturiz and Carbon 2000; Berild et al. 2008; Tunger et al. 2000).

Between 2003 and 2005, only 26% of all countries adopted a national strategy and less than half implemented public awareness and education programs (Khor 2005). This lack of action is of concern since:

1. The evidence that many chronic disorders are triggered by pathogens is mounting (Karin, Lawrence, and Nizet 2006).

2. It is feared that the spread of AMDR might worsen the outcomes for chronic and debilitating diseases of infectious origins, including cancers.

3. The safety of many medical and surgical technologically intensive procedures might be at risk of AMDR complications, including death.

In April 2005 WHO identified AMDR as one of the world's most pressing public health problems: "The problem is so serious that unless concerted action is taken worldwide, we run the risk of returning to the pre-antibiotic era when many more children than now died of infectious diseases and major surgery was impossible due to the risk of infection" (WHO 2005). The 2002–2003 WHO report on global prevalence of AMDR for select pathogens states that:

1. Malaria is chloroquine resistant in 81 out of 92 countries.

2. Up to 17% of tuberculosis cases are multi-drug resistant.

3. Up to 25% of HIV/AIDS cases are resistant to at least one first-line anti-retroviral drug.

4. Depending on the region, gonorrhea is 5–98% penicillin resistant worldwide and shows increasing resistance rates to fluoroquinolone.

5. Penicillin-resistant Streptococcus responsible for pneumonia and meningitis is affecting 70% patients in some countries.

6. Shigellosis is 10–90% ampicillin resistant and 5–95% trimethoprim/sulfamethoxazole resistant in many countries where diarrhea is endemic.

7. Staphylococcus aureus nosocomial infections are up to 70% resistant to all penicillins and cephalosporins.

In the fall of 2008, the World Medical Association (WMA) (WMA 2011), in response to the risk of an unraveling AMDR pandemic, updated its 1996 resolution on microbial resistance. This action was also co-sponsored by the American Medical Association (AMA). The School of Public Policy at George Mason University (SPP, GMU) contributed to the peer-review and update of the proposed resolution. The 2011 World

Health Day was marked on April 7, recognizing anti-microbial resistance, and HIV/AIDS drug resistance problems (WHO 2011). In February 2011, The Infectious Diseases Society of America issued updated guidelines for MRSA prevention and treatment (Liu et al. 2011). The 112th United States Congress is currently considering legislation intended to curtail the spread of AMDR while stimulating the development of new antibiotic drugs. Many European Union countries, Australia, Canada, and New Zealand have adopted some form of AMDR interventions (WHO 2009).

Finally the Editors would like to thank Dr. Tia Beritashvili for all her efforts in launching our Journal. She has begun a new career in medical policy research. We also would like to welcome our new Deputy Editor, Dr. Bonnie Stabile. She intends to maintain the highest standards in our publication. Dr. Stabile will share her expectations, ideas, and vision with the readership in the following issues of the Journal.

REFERENCES

Alanis, A.J. 2005. "Resistance to Antibiotics: Are We in the Post-Antibiotic Era?" *Archives of Medical Research* 36 (6): 697-705.

Awad, A., D.E. Ball, and I.B. Eltayeb. 2007. "Improving Rational Drug Use in Africa: the Example of Sudan." *Eastern Mediterranean Health Journal* 13 (5): 1202-1211.

Berild, D., T.G. Abrahamsen, S. Andresen, et al. 2008. "A Controlled Intervention Study to Improve Antibiotic Use in a Russian Pediatric Hospital." *International Journal of Antimicrobial Agents* 31 (5): 478-483.

Eurosurveillance. 2008. "Home." http://www.eurosurveillance.org/.

Higashi, T., and S. Furuhara. 2009. "Antibiotic Prescriptions for Upper Respiratory Tract Infection in Japan." *Internal Medicine* 48 (16): 1369-1375.

Holmberg, S.D., S.L. Solomon, and P.A. Blake. 1987. "Health and Economic Impacts of Antimicrobial Resistance." *Reviews of Infectious Diseases* 9 (6): 1065-1078.

Isturiz, R.E., and C. Carbon. 2000. "Antibiotic Use in Developing Countries." *Infection Control and Hospital Epidemiology* 21 (6): 394-397.

Kaier, K., C. Wilson, M. Chalkley, et al. 2008. "Health and Economic Impacts of Antibiotic Resistance in European Hospitals—Outlook on the BURDEN Project." *Infection* 36 (5): 492-494.

Karin, M., T. Lawrence, and V. Nizet. 2006. "Innate Immunity Gone Awry: Linking Microbial Infections to Chronic Inflammation and Cancer." *Cell* 124: 823-835.

Khor, M. 2005. "TWN Info Service on Health Issues No. 9—Irrational Drug Use Causing Rise of Anti-Microbial Resistance." *Third World Network.* www.twnside.org.sg/title2/health.info/twninfohealth009.htm.

Liu, C., A. Bayer, S.E. Cosgrove, et al. 2011. "Clinical Practice Guidelines by the Infectious Diseases Society of America for the Treatment of Methicillin-Resistant Staphylococcus Aureus Infections in Adults and Children: Executive Summary." Clinical Infectious Diseases 52 (3): 285-292.

Meropol, S.B., Z. Chen, and J.P. Metlay. 2009. "Reduced Antibiotic Prescribing for Acute Respiratory Infection in Adults and Children." British Journal of General Practice 59 (567): e321-e328.

Meyers, B.R. 1987. "Bacterial Resistance: Exploring the Facts and Myths." *Bulletin New York Academy of Medicine* 63 (3): 211-216.

PRWeb. 2011. "Global Antibiotics Market to Reach US$40.3 Billion by 2015, According to New Report by Global Industry Analysts, Inc." http://www.prweb.com/releases/antibiotics/anti_infectives/prweb4688824.htm.

Russell, A.D. 1997. "Plasmids and Bacterial Resistance to Biocides." *Journal of Applied Microbiology* 83 (2): 155-165.

Tucker, M.E. 2010. "Cost of Antibiotic Resistance Hits Private Payers." *Hospitalist News.* http://www.ehospitalistnews.com/specialty-focus/infectious-diseases/single-article-page/cost-of-antibiotic-resistance-hits-private-payers/6031fbf760.html.

Tunger, O., G. Dinc, B. Ozbakkaloglu, et al. 2000. "Evaluation of Rational Antibiotic Use." *International Journal of Antimicrobial Agents* 15 (2): 131-135.

Weinstein, R.A. 2001. "Controlling Antimicrobial Resistance in Hospitals: Infection Control and Use of Antibiotics." *Emerging Infectious Diseases* 7 (2): 188-192.

Woodward, R.S., G. Medoff, M.D. Smith, and J.L. Gray. 1987. "Antibiotic Cost Savings from Formulary Restrictions and Physician Monitoring in a Medical-School-Affiliated Hospital." *American Journal of Medicine* 83: 817-823.

World Health Organization (WHO). 2005. "Containing Antimicrobial Resistance." *WHO Policy Perspectives on Medicines.* http://www.who.int/management/anmicrobialresistance.pdf.

World Health Organization (WHO). 2009. "First Meeting of the WHO Advisory Group on Integrated Surveillance of Antimicrobial Resistance (AGISAR), June 15–19, 2009." http://www.who.int/foodborne_disease/resistance/agisar_June09/en/.

World Health Organization (WHO). 2010. "Medicines: Rational Use of Medicines." http://www.who.int/mediacentre/factsheets/fs338/en/index.html.

World Health Organization (WHO). 2011. "Home." http://whd2011.euro. who.int/.

World Medical Association (WMA). 2011. "WMA Statement on Resistance to Antimicrobial Drugs." http://www.wma.net/en/30publications/10policies/a19/index.html.

II.
INTERNATIONAL RESPONSES TO DISASTERS

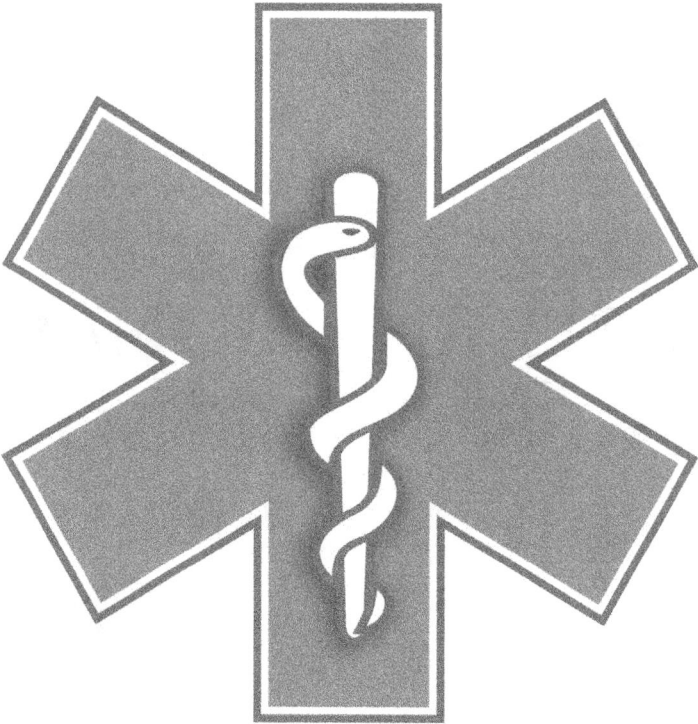

JAPAN MEDICAL ASSOCIATION'S ACTIONS IN THE GREAT EASTERN JAPAN EARTHQUAKE

Masami Ishii, *Japan Medical Association*
Takashi Nagata, *Japan Medical Association*
Katsuhito Aoki, *Japan Medical Association*

INTRODUCTION

The Great Eastern Japan Earthquake occurred in the Pacific Ocean off Japan's northeastern Sanriku coast at 14:46 JST on March 11, 2011, with a magnitude of 9.0. In the following six months, 199 aftershocks of magnitude 4 or greater occurred in the region (Nagamatsu et al. 2011). According to the national data from the National Police Agency, there were 15,811 deaths, 4,035 missing, and 5,932 severely injured (Table 1), and about 300,000 buildings were completely or partially destroyed by September 26 (National Police Agency 2011).

Table 1: Portrait of Patients in the Great Eastern Japan Earthquake and the Great Hanshin Earthquake

The main features of this disaster included the following: (1) widespread tsunami damage in Japan's northeastern Tohoku region across 500 km of the Pacific coastline; (2) the occurrence of a serious accident at the Fukushima Nuclear Power Plant; and (3) shortages of supplies and gasoline, which caused delayed distribution after disaster. Additionally, from the perspective of healthcare providers, the following phenomena were noted: (1) dysfunction of numerous hospitals, clinics, and welfare facilities for older people due to tsunami damage; (2) many fatalities caused by drowning immediately after the tsunami, with limited numbers of severe injuries; (3) a high need for autopsies of disaster casualties in the early stages of the disaster; (4) occupation of evacuation shelters for months by evacuees and survivors; and (5) a high proportion (>30%) of individuals aged 65 years and older in disaster-affected areas, with a pre-existing shortage of physicians.

Additionally, handling of the Fukushima nuclear accident, particularly delayed disclosure of information by the government and Tokyo Electric Power Company (TEPCO), caused a serious problem. The government issued an evacuation order for those living within a 20-km radius of Fukushima Daiichi Nuclear Power Plant (Daiichi) on March 12; however, evacuation of areas outside this 20-km radius was delayed because information was not properly disclosed. As a consequence, social fear was exaggerated and many people fled Fukushima, having a serious impact on the recovery of the region (Ishii 2011a; 2011c).

Table 2: Status of JMAT/JMAT II Operations

JMAT (activites ended on July 15)	
	Teams dispatched
Iwate Prefecture	398
JMAT Iwate	56
Miyagi Prefecture	643
Fukushima Prefecture	272
Ibaraki Prefecture	12
*JMATs that were dispatched to several prefectures	3
Total	1,384

JMAT II (from July 16)		
	In action**	On stanby
Iwate Prefecture (including JMAT Iwate)	81	10
Miyagi Prefecture	52	6
Fukushima Prefecture	27	11
Total	160	27

** includes those whose dispatch has been settled.
(as of Sep 22)

Table 2: Status of JMAT/JMAT II Operations

THE JAPAN MEDICAL ASSOCIATION AND JAPAN MEDICAL ASSISTANCE TEAMS (JMATS)

The Japan Medical Association (JMA), with 165,000 members, is a professional association for physicians and also Japan's largest non-governmental organization (NGO) (Ishii et al. 2010). The mission of the JMA is to improve and maintain the healthcare system in Japan through its own code of conduct and professional autonomy (World Medical Association 2008). At the same time, JMA ensures cooperation with the government (Ishii, Hamamoto, and Tsuruoka 2010).

The JMA recognized the importance of disaster preparedness upon hosting the World Medical Association's 2006 Asian-Pacific Regional Conference in Tokyo, where the main topics were pandemic flu and earthquake/tsunami preparation (Chun 2007; Tsuji 2007; Yamamoto 2007). This event spurred the creation of the Japan Medical Association Teams (JMATs).

95

JMATs are the medical assistance teams organized by JMA members to respond to all kinds of health crises (described in detail later). These teams differ somewhat from the government's Disaster Medical Assistance Teams (DMATs), established in 2005 (Kondo et al. 2009). DMATs are deployed to the scene immediately (48–72 hours) following a disaster, especially those with mass causalities, to provide triage, treatment, and transfer for individuals with severe injuries. JMATs, on the other hand, administer medical relief in both acute and chronic phases following a disaster. However, while DMATs focus on trauma and critical patients, JMATs perform a variety of medical/public health work for people in disaster-affected areas.

Following the Great Eastern Japan Earthquake, DMATs were deployed in the super-acute phase. Although they demonstrated an ability to mobilize quickly, they were unable to fulfill their primary mission because of a limited number of severe injuries (Ishii 2011b; 2011c). JMATs were also deployed following this disaster—the first deployment of such teams by the JMA's activities composed the core of the JMA disaster response to the Great Eastern Japan Earthquake, and 1,384 teams with members having diverse clinical backgrounds were dispatched by July 15, 2011.

The JMA's disaster response extended beyond providing healthcare to disaster survivors through JMATs. In addition to JMAT deployment, the JMA conducted many operations to support and restore the healthcare system in the disaster-affected areas in the short, medium, and long term. Further, because of Japan's risk for future natural disasters—earthquake, tsunami, volcanic eruption, typhoon, etc.—in addition to the social issues of rapidly aging societies, undistributed and too few physicians, and an overused universal health insurance system—all issues revealed after the disaster—the JMA recognizes that much remains to be addressed from the standpoint of healthcare providers.

JMAT OPERATIONS

JMAT/JMAT II Overview

JMATs are DMATs that, upon request from the JMA, are formed and dispatched from prefectural medical associations based on requests from the prefectural medical association of a disaster-affected area (Ishii 2011a; 2011b; 2011c). The mission statement and the number of deployed teams and the background of team members deployed following the "3.11" disaster are described in Tables 2, 3, and 4, respectively. Initial JMATs, 1,384 in total, were dispatched by July 15. After JMAT withdrawal based on local requests, JMAT II was deployed. All JMAT members were registered by the JMA, and travel insurance was guaranteed. Also, the JMAT field activity costs were reimbursed by the government.

Because a wide area of eastern Japan was damaged, the JMA assigned JMATs from all of Japan to the four disaster-affected prefectures (Iwate, Miyagi, Fukushima, and Ibaraki), and coordinated their deployment as efficiently as possible. In field activities, JMATs used the evacuation shelter evaluation sheets (Table 5) and triage cards to collect updated field information. Triage cards contain three color-coded categories: red for sick patients needing medical care, yellow for stable patients needing regular prescriptions, and white for evacuees without medical conditions (Figure 1). These triage cards were important as they ensured efficient transfer of medical information between teams.

Figure 1: JMAT Triage Card

The main purpose of JMAT II is to prevent disaster-associated morbidities and mortality in the long term, including mental health issues and solitary deaths, and providing healthcare visits at temporary housing, etc. JMAT II operations also included providing support to areas or hospitals facing a serious shortage of physicians and other healthcare workers. Because disaster survivors initially stayed in evacuation shelters and then slowly moved to temporary housing, long-term healthcare support was mandatory. In contrast to JMATs, whose costs are reimbursed by the government because of the nature of their work as disaster relief, JMAT II operates within the normal healthcare setting, and its costs are covered by the universal health insurance system.

Occupation	Total
Physician*	2,150
Nurse, Assistant nurse	1,681
Pharmacist	445
Coordination staff	1,084
Other**	481
Total	5,841

(as of Aug 11, 2011)

*Out of all the physicians who registered in the JMAT scheme, JMA members accounted for 60%, almost the same composition as the JMA's memership ratio. This shows how physicians from across the country came together.

**The Other category includes physical therapists, occupational therapists, clinical laboratory technicians, clinical radiologists, social workers, psychiatric social workers, clinical psychologists, care managers, and nutritionists, etc.

Table 4: Number of JMAT/JMAT II Participants by Type of Occupation

These checklists were prepared by the Japan Medical Association following the Great Eastern Japan Earthquake to be used by JMATs for making simple activity records and for handing over duties to successor teams.

Prepared by: _____ of the _____ Medical Association
Date prepared:
Shelter name:
Shelter address:
Capacity:
Gender ratio:
Vulnerable people (elderly, children, pregnant women, dialysis patients, determination of treatment necessity):
Medical needs (including sufficiency of drugs):
Possibility of radiation exposure:
Water/food
Toilet/hygiene:
Persons needing nursing care:
No. of JMAT Evacuation Center Triage Cards: Red   , Yellow   White
Other:

Table 5 Items included in the JMAT Evacuation Center Checklist

JMAT Timeline—Before the Disaster to the Dispatch

Creation of JMATs was proposed by the JMA's Committee on Emergency and Disaster Medicine in March 2010 (Ishii 2011b). When the disaster occurred, JMATs were still under development, with debate about their primary mission and appropriate training courses. Several disaster training courses were proposed, including the American Medical Association's National Disaster Life Support (NDLS) program (Coule and Schwartz 2009) or the DMAT curriculum as a standard for the JMA concept.

Four days after the earthquake, the JMA decided to dispatch JMATs. The primary mission of JMATs was established as medical and public health support in evacuation shelters from the acute phase, in addition to primary care and autopsies in large-scale disasters.

Once JMATs were deployed, the JMA regularly and carefully considered the needs for these teams in the disaster-affected areas with the local prefectural medical associations (Iwate, Miyagi, Fukushima, and Ibaraki). Because of reduced medical needs, the JMA decided to stop dispatching teams to Ibaraki on March 24. Subsequently, JMA leaders visited those three prefectural medical associations in Iwate, Miyagi, and Fukushima, on April 14, and decided to continue sending teams. The healthcare system in the disaster-affected areas gradually recovered; thus the need for outside support decreased. On June 28, JMA decided to deploy all JMATs by July 15 to the disaster-affected areas. However, in some areas, continuous support was mandatory because of delayed healthcare recovery, and JMAT II was dispatched after July 15. The activity of JMATs is disaster relief work, and its costs are reimbursed by the government, while JMAT II works in the normal healthcare setting and its costs are covered by the universal health insurance system.

JMAT Activities and Challenges

Lessons from the JMA response to the 3.11 disaster must be integrated and used to prepare for the next disaster. JMA is currently reviewing JMAT field activities and considering future disaster relief plans. An appropriate training course must be implemented; training will be counted as continuing medical education (CME) programs for JMAT participants and JMA members. The disaster cycle of JMAT is shown in Figure 2.

a. Pre-disaster phase:

- providing disaster medical education and training for JMA members and JMAT participants;
- conducting disaster vulnerability assessment and creating a disaster plan accordingly;
- participation of the national and prefectural disaster management administration meeting;
- communicating with diverse relevant organizations and groups to establish mutual aid in case of disaster;
- developing a disaster management system for medical institutions nationwide, and preparing hospital ships and air ambulances for disaster.

b. Disaster response phase (JMAT dispatch):

- deploying JMATs according to the request of disaster-affected areas;
- transporting medical supplies as needed;
- sharing information with other disaster organizations such as DMATs, Japan Red Cross, etc.

c. Healthcare support for disaster survivors (JMAT maintenance and withdrawal):

- managing disaster survivors' health at home, in shelters, and in temporary housing;

- transferring tasks from JMATs to local medical providers, such as medical/public health support needs in evacuation shelters, recovery of the local medical institutions, etc.;
- cooperating with other professionals operating in the disaster-affected areas (e.g., public health nurses, nutritionists, caregivers, and welfare providers);
- withdrawing JMATs according to the progress of healthcare restoration in the disaster-affected areas.

d. Recovery phase (healthcare restoration):
  - securing public finance support for healthcare in the disaster-affected areas;
  - ensuring countermeasures for post-traumatic stress disorder for JMAT participants.

PRIMARY JMA ACTIONS IN THE FIRST MONTH FOLLOWING THE 3.11 DISASTER

a. Immediately after the earthquake occurred on March 11, the JMA set up the Disaster Countermeasures Headquarters, led by the President. Staffed by other JMA administrators, this headquarters functioned 24 hours a day, 7 days a week in the first month. Many officers as well as researchers from the JMA Research Institute conducted field inspections and conferred with the medical associations of the disaster-affected prefectures and local health personnel toward the goal of meeting future medical needs and rebuilding the community health structure in afflicted areas.

b. Transportation of a large amount of medical supplies on March 19 with support from the U.S. military and Embassy and Japan Self-Defense Forces (JSDF). In fact, 8.5-ton truckloads of drugs were sent to Iwate and Miyagi. At the same time, the Aichi Medical Association transported medical supplies to Fukushima by a Mitsubishi Heavy Industries private jet. These supplies have been used effectively by mobilized JMATs in addition to local physicians. Staff from the Harvard Humanitarian Initiatives worked as a liaison for both Japan and the United States. From the standpoint of humanitarian support, the U.S. embassy facilitated the U.S. military, and, for the U.S. military, this operation was one of the initial successes in Operation Tomodachi, the joint operation of the United States and Japan to support disaster relief.

c. The majority of fatalities in this earthquake disaster were caused by drowning soon after the tsunami. Autopsy for disaster casualties and burials of those individuals were important. The National Police Agency asked JMA to send experienced physicians for autopsy. The JMA had previously established cooperation with the Japanese Academic Society for Forensic Physicians; such connections allowed the JMA to recruit physicians for this mission.

d. Immediately after the disaster, JMA distributed the latest information to JMA members and the public via JMA's website and faxes. This information included surveillance mapping of the radiation measurements in Fukushima (Ishii 2011a).

e. DMAT activities ended on March 27, which was longer than the original field activity period (72 hours). Because the needs of healthcare and public health support for evacuation shelters were prolonged, JMATs were required to continue the deployment for a longer time.

f. Power plant shutdowns, including the Fukushima Daiichi Nuclear Power Plant accident, resulted in electric power shortages in the Tokyo metropolitan area, where TEPCO creates a monopoly on electricity. Rolling blackouts were implemented between March 14 and 27. JMA strongly protested these measures and advocated for the provision of electricity to medical institutions and to patients requiring at-home medical care, including respirators.

g. The shortage of gasoline caused by the effects of the earthquake was a major obstacle in sending JMATs and other medical teams into the field. The JMA president contacted the Minister of Land, Infrastructure and Transport directly, and requested the prioritizing of gasoline supply to medical personnel.

h. The JMA negotiated with the domestic airline companies for the provision of free air transport for JMATs.

OTHER DISASTER RELIEF-ASSOCIATED MISSIONS
OF THE JMA IN SUB-ACUTE PHASE

a. The JMA launched the Disaster Survivors Health Support Liaison Council comprising 34 healthcare organizations as well as the government's Cabinet Office and the Ministries of Health, Labor and Welfare; Education; Culture, Sports, Science and Technology; and Internal Affairs and Communications. The Council discusses the needs of the disaster-affected areas. The JMA wishes to continue meetings of the Council once the disaster situation returns to normal to ensure that medical/public health support for disaster survivors is instituted efficiently following future disasters.

b. The JMA started collecting donations from across the country soon after the earthquake. The total amount of donations reached 1.9 billion yen by August 31, 2011. The entire sum was sent to medical associations in the disaster-affected areas.

c. The JMA negotiated with the government and the Democratic Party for health management of disaster survivors and restoration of the healthcare system in the disaster-affected areas. Further, the JMA requested the creation of a fund to be utilized not only for urgent support but over the medium to long term. The JMA also requested financial support for private clinic physicians burdened by loans for their clinics. In preparation for future disasters, the JMA requested the construction of hospital ships to service disaster areas. In Fukushima, many healthcare workers fled for fear of radiation exposure from the Daiichi Nuclear Power Plant incident; the JMA requested the government to use the financial support flexibly for employees' payment.

d. The JMA established the Project Team Committee for Recovery from the Fukushima Nuclear Accident. The Committee supports the reimbursement of JMA members who suffered damage from the Fukushima Daiichi Nuclear Power Plant accident. Additionally, relevant parties and the International Association of Emergency Managers (IAEM) donated radioactive substance decontamination gel to the Fukushima Medical

Association. On August 3, decontamination using this gel was demonstrated at a kindergarten in Fukushima.

e. In this disaster, numerous medical institutions, including prefectural hospitals that were cores of their local communities, were washed away by the tsunami. The JMA donated a temporary medical clinic to replace services provided by one such hospital, Iwate Prefectural Otsuchi Hospital. Additionally, a number of trailer houses were provided as temporary medical clinics.

f. The JMA urged medical institutions outside the disaster-affected areas to prescribe small amounts of medication to patients so that the limited supply of medicines would be available to disaster areas. The JMA also initiated public health promotion to secure sanitation/hygiene in evacuation shelters to protect vulnerable people. Additionally, the distribution of both automated external defibrillators and the Japan Geriatrics Society's Manual of Medical Care for the Elderly during a Disaster to evacuation shelters was achieved through the JMA.

FUKUSHIMA DAIICHI NUCLEAR ACCIDENT AND THE JMA

On March 11, the Fukushima Daiichi Nuclear Power Plant (Daiichi) lost power for the reactor cooling system as a result of earthquake and tsunami damage. Hydrogen explosions followed at Reactor 1 on March 12 and at Reactor 3 on March 14, triggering explosions and fires at Reactors 2 and 4 on March 15. In an attempt to control the situation, on March 17 helicopters from the Japan Self Defense Force poured tons of water on the reactors. The next day Fire Rescue Teams were deployed to establish a water supply system for cooling. On March 19, TEPCO connected the electricity from outside electrical lines and restored the cooling system for the reactors. After March 20, the situation at Daiichi began to improve gradually.

After the critical accident at the Tokai nuclear fuel plant in 1999, the Nuclear Safety Research Association established a network of radiation emergency medicine in prefectures with nuclear plants. A regional network was formed in the Department of Radiology at Fukushima Medical University. A network of primary care facilities in the vicinity was developed; Fukushima Medical University was designated as the secondary medical care institution, while the National Institute of Radiological Sciences was designated as the tertiary medical care institution for eastern Japan. However, many hospitals in Fukushima did not participate in this network prior to 3.11. Importantly, several hospitals near the Fukushima Daiichi Nuclear Power Plant and local medical association members had taken radiation emergency medicine training and had participated in annual emergency drills voluntarily.

After the accident at the Daiichi Plant, three medical institutions designated as primary radiation emergency medicine facilities and the off-site center that should have served as a command center in an emergency could not function at all. The reason is because all these facilities were located within 3–5 km from Daiichi and, in the situation following the explosions, the evacuation order was given to these areas. The initial response by Fukushima Medical University also could not work well because of confusion. Additionally, the backup command center located in the city of Minamisoma could not work due to earthquake damage. On March 11 and 12, medical response for Daiichi was completely out of control because of lack of information, command, and leadership. Additionally, the result of System for Prediction of Environmental Emergency Dose Information (SPEEDI), which is used to predict the distribution of radiation by computer simulation soon after the incident, was not disclosed, and evacuation was delayed.

Around March 13, many radiation emergency medicine experts from all over Japan, including from the Nuclear Safety Research Association, the National Institute of Radiological Sciences, Hiroshima University, and Nagasaki University, went to Fukushima for support, and gradually the Headquarters of Fukushima Prefecture took the initiative.

The city of Iwaki, which is located 40 km south of the Daiichi Plant, is the second largest city (population: 350,000) in the northeastern Tohoku region. It suffered tremendous damage along the coast due to the earthquake and tsunami. In addition, Iwaki city accepted residents who had evacuated from municipalities near Daiichi. On March 13, there were about 20,000 evacuees in 150 evacuation shelters in the city.

Following the disaster, the president and vice president of the local Iwaki Medical Association and local medical institutions immediately began disaster medical operations to support evacuees in the shelters and disaster survivors. JMAT members from the JMA joined this mission from March 13. However, subsequent explosions at Daiichi and the government's inappropriate response led to serious social fear and distrust; daily necessities such as water, food, medical supplies, and gasoline were not delivered at all. On March 15, the city was in a chaotic situation, and disaster medical support operations had to be temporarily suspended. On March 17, the U.S. government prohibited its citizens from entering a zone within an 80-km radius around Daiichi. At the same time, the JMA analyzed the actual conditions of radiation exposure in Fukushima Prefecture and Iwaki city. The analysis results showed that the distribution of radioactive contamination was shifting to the north-west area from Daiichi by wind and weather, rather than in concentric circles as presented by the government. Also, the measurement of radiation in most areas in Fukushima on March 17 was within 1 μSv per hour, which was thought to be critical for acute radiation syndrome. On March 18, JMA made the decision to send JMATs to the cities in Fukushima (Ishii 2011a). With the cooperation of local healthcare workers and JMATs, the situation of evacuees in the shelters of Fukushima became stable, and the appearance of medical teams outside reassured everyone. Thereafter, local medical institutions were gradually restored, and JMAT deployment was gradually reduced. Iodine tablets were distributed to all houses within 20 km from Daiichi, and people waited for instructions to take them. On March 18, Iwaki city Mayor decided to distribute iodine tablets to 300,000 people according to the request of the Iwaki Medical Association. On the other hand, the national government never ordered the tablets intake.

By the end of May, most cities in Fukushima could close the medical support operations, including JMATs, and the situation became almost normal. Currently, Iwaki city, following the critical situation in March at Daiichi, is in the midst of an economic boom and embracing about 5,000 workers to restore Daiichi.

Since June, the JMA has started several medical support actions through the Survivors Health Support Liaison Council and through the Project Committee for Recovery from the Fukushima Nuclear Accident.

SPECIAL CONSIDERATIONS OF THE HEALTHCARE SYSTEM IN JAPAN ASSOCIATED WITH DISASTER RESPONSE

Shortage and Uneven Distribution of Physicians and Nurses in Japan

The shortage of physicians in Japan has become a major social problem in recent years, with only 2.15 clinicians per 1,000 people in Japan in 2008—one of the lowest among the Organisation for Economic Co-operation and Development (OECD) countries (OECD 2011). Further, the number of physicians per population varies widely across prefectures in Japan. The government has tried to resolve this shortage by increasing the number of medical schools and medical students per school. While this countermeasure might be effective in the long term, it does not help the current situation. Additionally, a similar problem is observed for nurses. According to the Ministry of Health, Labor, and Welfare, the shortage of nursing personnel will rise from 14,900 in 2011 to 56,000 in 2015 (Ministry of Health, Labor and Welfare 2010). Adding to these shortages, the government intends to reduce the number of hospitals and hospital beds to alleviate a budget shortfall (Ishii, Hamamoto, and Tsuruoka 2010). Thus, the surge of patients during the 3.11 disaster overwhelmed the healthcare system. The main disaster-affected areas after 3.11 were places with especially limited medical resources; there is concern that this situation might be exacerbated by the loss of medical institutions and the deaths of and by the drain of healthcare workers to other places. Unfortunately, such a problem may not be restricted to Japan: healthcare worker shortages in other nations may lead to similar situations in the future.

Japan's Disaster Medical System

In the Great Hanshin Earthquake of January 17, 1995, more than 6,000 were killed and more than 10,000 were severely injured (Table 1). The medical response to these severe/fatal disaster injuries was not conducted appropriately (Kondo et al. 2009). On the basis of this experience, a disaster medical response system, including DMATs, was created. DMAT members receive specialized training and have the mobility to operate during the acute phase of a disaster (generally within the first 48 hours). They are included in the national government's Master Plan for Disaster Management. However, DMATs do not cover healthcare support for evacuees in shelters or offer mental health or public health support and other medical works necessary over the long term. One of JMAT's missions is to fulfill this role, and it was quite meaningful in this disaster.

Japan's location near the Pacific Rim areas encircling the Pacific Ocean places it at high risk for future natural disasters. Thus, preparation for future disaster is absolutely mandatory, and the system should be revised according to the lessons learned from the Great Eastern Japan Earthquake.

Vulnerable Groups (Especially Older Persons)

During disaster, especially in cases of mass casualty incidents, emergency medical care for trauma/burn/critical patients is the highest priority. However, vulnerable groups such as those aged 65 years and older, children, pregnant women, and people with special care (hemodialysis, etc.) can be defined as a high-risk population for disaster-related morbidity and mortality. Japan has a rapidly aging population by international comparison. The number of people aged 65 years or older was about 29 million in 2009, accounting for 22.8% of the total population, and is estimated to reach 30.5% in 2025 (The National Institute of Population and Social Security Research 2010). Moreover, in 2010 there were 15.7 million households with a person over the age of 64 years, accounting for 31.2% overall. Among those households, 5,336,000 consisted of couples only, and 4,665,000 consisted of an older person living alone (Cabinet Office, Japan 2010). Additionally, patients who need hemodialysis are increasing annually in Japan, with a total of 297,216 people receiving continuous hemodialysis in December 2010 (Japanese Society for Dialysis Therapy 2011). Following the 3.11 disaster, there were difficulties in providing healthcare and evacuating these vulnerable people, especially older persons and patients receiving continuous hemodialysis.

Evacuation Shelters and Dying a Solitary Death

It is relatively common for evacuees, including older persons, to live in shelters in groups over long periods, even in industrialized countries. Most evacuation shelters are public facilities such as school gymnasiums, public halls, etc. Evacuees must sleep on the floor, basic supplies such as water, food, and electricity are not always adequate, and individual privacy is not guaranteed. Evacuees suffer from worsening sanitary conditions, emotional stress, loss of sleep, and fatigue. Following the Great Eastern Japan Earthquake, nearly 400,000 people were evacuated at the peak. Gradually, evacuees were moved to temporary housing; however, even three months after the disaster, there were still about 90,000 people living in evacuation shelters.

Older individuals are at a relatively high risk of solitary death, dying alone at their residences, in evacuation shelters, or in temporary housing. In shelters, older people stay with others; however, once moved to temporary housing, they tend to be separated and isolated. These conditions might accelerate solitary death (Fujita et al. 2008), and local healthcare workers are very concerned about preventing this problem.

CONCLUSION

The Great Eastern Japan Earthquake caused extensive and widespread damage, also triggering a nuclear accident that fostered social fear and distrust. The JMA fulfilled its social mission for evacuees and patients in disaster-affected areas with the cooperation of many organizations and various healthcare workers. As Japan is faced with many natural disaster risks, such as earthquakes, tsunamis, and volcanic eruptions, and has numerous nuclear power plants and chemical complexes, better disaster response plans are mandatory. Using lessons learned from the Great Eastern Japan Earthquake, the JMA analyzed JMAT operations in this disaster retrospectively, and will provide disaster medicine training as part of CME programs and strengthen the disaster preparedness of the healthcare system at national, prefectural, and local levels.

Figure 2: JMA's Actions during a Disaster and Disaster Preparedness

POLICY IMPLICATIONS

Healthcare professionals worldwide have a social obligation to prepare for disasters. Medical relief work, especially for large-scale disasters, should cover not only trauma and critical care in the acute phase, but also healthcare for evacuees in shelters, autopsy, mental health follow-up, and restoration of the healthcare system in disaster-affected areas. Also, preparation for nuclear accidents, including radiation emergency medicine, is mandatory.

REFERENCES

Cabinet Office, Japan. 2010. "Annual Report on the Aging Society." www8.cao.go.jp/kourei/whitepaper/w-2010/zenbun/pdf/1s2s_1_1.pdf (accessed November 17, 2011).

Chun, S.D. 2007. "The Experiences from KMA's Recent Activities." *The Japan Medical Association Journal* 50 (1): 80-88.

Coule, P.L., and R.B. Schwartz. 2009. "The National Disaster Life Support Programs: A Model for Competency-Based Standardized and Locally Relevant Training." Journal of Public Health Management and Practice 15 (2 Suppl.): S25-S30.

Fujita, Y., K. Inoue, N. Seki, T. Inoue, A. Sakuta, T. Miyazawa, and K. Eguchi. 2008. "The Need for Measures to Prevent 'Solitary deaths' After Large Earthquakes—Based on Current Conditions following the Great Hanshin-Awaji Earthquake." *Journal of Forensic and Legal Medicine* 15 (8): 527-528.

Ishii, M. 2011a. "Fukushima Nuclear Power Plant Accidents Caused by Gigantic Earthquake and Tsunami –Healthcare Support for Radiation Exposure." *The World Medical Journal* 57 (4): 141-144.

Ishii, M. 2011b. "Japan Medical Association Team's (JMAT) First Call to Action in the Great Eastern Japan Earthquake." *The Japan Medical Association Journal* 54 (3): 144-154.

Ishii, M. 2011c. "Japan Medical Association Team's (JMATs) First Operation: Responding to the Great Eastern Japan Earthquake." *The World Medical Journal* 57 (4): 131-140.

Ishii M., M. Hamamoto, and H. Tsuruoka. 2010. "JMA Perspectives on the Universal Health Insurance System in Japan." *The Japan Medical Association Journal* 53 (3): 139-143.

Japanese Society for Dialysis Therapy. 2011. "An Overview of Regular Dialysis Treatment in Japan of December 31, 2010." http://docs.jsdt.or.jp/overview/pdf2011/p08.pdf (in Japanese. accessed November 17, 2011).

Kondo, H., Y. Koido, K. Morino, M. Homma, Y. Otomo, Y. Yamamoto, and H. Henmi. 2009. "Establishing Disaster Medical Assistance Teams in Japan." *Prehospital and Disaster Medicine* 24 (6): 556-564.

Ministry of Health, Labor and Welfare, Japan. 2010. "Seventh Supply and Demand Outlook for Nursing Staffs in Japan." www.mhlw.go.jp/stf/houdou/2r9852000000z68f-img/2r9852000000z6df.pdf (accessed November 17, 2011).

Nagamatsu, S., T. Maekawa, Y. Ujike, S. Hashimoto, and N. Fuke, Japanese Society of Intensive Care. 2011. "The Earthquake and Tsunami—Observations by Japanese Physicians Since the 11 March Catastrophe." Critical Care 15 (3): 167.

National Police Agency. 2011. "Damage Situation and Police Countermeasures Associated with 2011 Tohoku District—Off the Pacific Ocean Earthquake October 7, 2011." http://www.npa.go.jp/archive/keibi/biki/higaijokyo.pdf (accessed November 17, 2011).

Organization for Economic Co-Operation and Development. 2011. "OECD Health Data 2011." http://stats.oecd.org/index.aspx?DataSetCode=HEALTH_STAT (accessed November 17, 2011).

The National Institute of Population and Social Security Research. 2010. "Population Statistics of Japan 2008." http://www.ipss.go.jp/ (accessed November 17, 2011).

Tsuji, Y. 2007. "Mechanism of the Occurrence of Earthquakes and Tsunamis." The Japan Medical Association Journal 50 (1): 55-71.

World Medical Association. 2008. "WMA Declaration of Seoul on Professional Autonomy and Clinical Independence." www.wma.net/en/30publications/10policies/a30/ (accessed November 17, 2011).

Yamamoto, Y. 2007. "Disaster Management in the Acute Phase." *The Japan Medical Association Journal* 50 (1): 72-79.

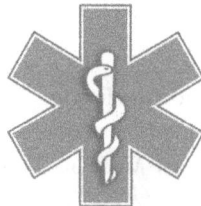

VOLUNTEERED GEOGRAPHIC INFORMATION AND CROWDSOURCING DISASTER RELIEF: A CASE STUDY OF THE HAITIAN EARTHQUAKE

Matthew Zook, PhD, *University of Kentucky*
Mark Graham, PhD, *University of Oxford*
Taylor Shelton, BA, *University of Kentucky*
Sean Gorman, PhD, *FortiusOne*

INTRODUCTION

"Is that road up there passable? . . . Does it really exist?"
—*(Wohltman 2010)*

When the magnitude 7.0 earthquake struck Haiti on January 12, 2010, there was an immediate need for maps. Emergency responders had to know where the people most in need were located and how to get assistance and relief to them. Large parts of Haiti and its capital, Port-au-Prince, lacked adequate coverage in the standard web mapping services (e.g., Bing Maps and Google Maps) that people in most of the developed world have grown accustomed to using. As one of the world's poorest countries, Haiti had simply not provided the kind of demand for online mapping that drove its expansion elsewhere. Post-earthquake, the demand for spatial information and online maps increased tremendously and, given the urgency of relief operations, the ability to crowdsource the data collection process became particularly important.

This paper outlines some of the ways in which information technologies (ITs) were used in the Haiti relief effort, especially with respect to web-based mapping services. It demonstrates that ITs were a key means through which individuals could make a tangible difference in the work of relief and aid agencies without actually being physically present in Haiti. While not without problems, this effort nevertheless represents a remarkable example of the power of crowdsourced online mapping and the potential for new avenues of interaction between physically distant places.

The first section of this paper briefly reviews the history of IT, mapping, and disaster response with a particular focus on the role of volunteered data acquisition and distribution. The second part of the paper reviews some of the key ICT infrastructures employed during the Haitian earthquake crisis. Finally, the paper discusses potential lessons from the experience of crowdsourcing and disaster relief. While these lessons are preliminary and best viewed as a starting point rather than a final format, the earthquake in Chile on February 27, 2010, reiterates the importance and relevance of these efforts.

Mapping Disasters

> *"It is sobering to be reminded that one of the basic instincts of human nature—mutual cooperation for no cost—is thriving on a global scale." (Keegan 2010)*

Natural and anthropogenic disasters have occurred throughout history, and the trappings of the twenty-first century (e.g., global climate change, population growth, spread of infectious disease) seem to indicate that they will surely continue. Responses to disasters, however, have changed both in people's sense of connection to distance places and in their ability to contribute to relief efforts. Both these changes are strongly tied to ITs, which have long allowed for the broadcasting of news about disasters in a one-to-many fashion, but are now beginning to allow people to respond directly to these disasters by way of a many-to-many model.

IT and Disaster Response

For the most part, research on disaster response has assumed that states or other quasi-governmental entities (e.g., the United Nations) would be the primary actors in disaster relief, with nongovernmental organizations (NGOs) playing a secondary role. Therefore it comes as no surprise that the role of IT was primarily viewed as a means to enhance the command, control, and dissemination of information (Alexander 1991; Comfort 1993; Gruntfest and Weber 1998; Quarantelli 1997). Much of the early research focused primarily on the positive side of IT in disaster recovery (Alexander 1991), although later research also recognized the complications within command structures resulting from nonproximate technology use (Stephenson and Anderson 1997). Questions were also raised as to whether disaster response plans incorporating IT only mirror non-IT disaster response plans, and whether these plans are even put into practice in the event of a disaster (Fischer 1998). But in almost all cases there was little thought given to the role of individuals or ad hoc networks emerging in response to the crisis.

Despite this tendency, some research has also focused on the variety of ways that telecommunications (including personal and individual exchanges) are a vital part of disaster response and can help mitigate losses and personal trauma (Townsend and Moss 2005). In addition to the importance at the individual level of the continuity of communication, others have examined how these ITs can empower activists and citizens on the ground during crises to work for the public good (Fischer 1999; Rodrigue 2001). Moreover, the past three decades have seen an ideological shift away from the state and emphasizing the importance of the market or private forces (e.g., neoliberalism) in regulating society (Harvey 2005). If nothing else, the quasi-ubiquitous web of personal communication can lead to serious rethinking of how the state (at a range of scales) should provide early warning and response to disasters (Rodriguez et al. 2007).

115

The Rise of Web 2.0 and Mapping

Concurrent with this shift of emphasis from the role of IT in state-led disaster response is the growing significance of what is often referred to as Web 2.0. Also referred to as peer production, cloud collaboration, or cloud sourcing, the phenomenon refers to the ability of people from around the world to collaborate on projects that are often highly ambitious in both their scale and scope (Graham 2010a). It also marks the "...increased ability for individual users and loosely affiliated networks to construct and shape cyberspace and their daily lives" (Crutcher and Zook 2009, 524).

By 2006, it was recognized that the peer production of information had become so transformational that Time magazine voted "you" (that is, creators of user-generated content) as their person of the year, with the editor arguing that Web 2.0 represents nothing short of a revolution because it is no longer "the few, the powerful and the famous who shape our collective destiny as a species" (Grossman 2006). One prime example of Web 2.0 style mapping is the OpenStreetMap (OSM) project, which leverages Global Positioning System (GPS) trails and digitized street patterns from aerial imagery to create a free street map for the entire world. Although developed countries enjoy better coverage than poor countries, the OSM project proved to be an important source of Web 2.0 mapping during the Haitian crisis.

What drives millions of people around the world to contribute their labor for free? Research has shown that the gift economy is often driven both by participants' desires to gain cultural capital by sharing and creating information and by a widespread desire to help other people (for example, in the case of medical bloggers) (Karimi and Poo 2009; Kollock 1999; Preece and Shneiderman 2009). The desire of participants to gain technical knowledge and see their contributions as a rewarding educational experience has also been identified as an important factor behind contributions to crowdsourced projects and virtual communities (Holohan and Garg 2005; Lakhani and von Hippel 2003).

The peer production of information has reshaped a variety of practices, but arguably none as profoundly as the production of geographic information where many users have moved from being passive recipients of geographic information to being producers themselves (Budhathoki, Bruce, and Nedovic-Budic 2008). A core motivation behind the production of volunteered geographic information (VGI) is likely the inaccessibility and cost of accurate sources of geographic information (Haklay and Weber 2008). The capacity of people from around the world to create geographic information has further been assisted by the drop in the price of GPS units and the wide availability of computers (Graham 2010b; Haklay and Weber 2008). Finally, the desire simply to fill in the blank spaces on the map and reveal the previously hidden should not be underestimated as a factor behind participation (Goodchild 2007; Perkins and Dodge 2008; Sui 2008).

Web 2.0 and Disaster Mapping

With the aforementioned development of OpenStreetMap (OSM) and a variety of other web-based mapping services (such as Google Maps), the ability for volunteers to assist in disaster response situations via mapping and other spatial analysis has grown significantly. Given the immediate need for reliable maps in volatile disaster response situations, the model of peer produced mapping provides a number of new avenues for producing and accessing spatial data, apart from the traditional models of top-down geographic information system (GIS) provision. This new constellation of social and technological forces provides a number of benefits, yet also faces shortcomings.

Perhaps the greatest benefit to this form of distributed mapping is that a greater number of maps can be produced in a shorter period of time, allowing scarce technical resources to be diverted elsewhere. This is especially the case for labor, as volunteer, crowdsourced mapping allows aid agencies to focus their limited resources on other needs that cannot be so easily met via distributed, volunteer workers.

A second important benefit of Web 2.0 and disaster mapping is the ability to leverage ITs to allow individuals to report on local and specific conditions. These uses come in a wide range of forms, including name-based databases that allow reports on or searches for individuals such as Google's Haitian Earthquake Person Finder (http:// haiticrisis.appspot.com/). Other examples include the Scipionus map following the Hurricane Katrina disaster, which allowed users to tie comments about local conditions, e.g., "there was three feet of water here," to specific locations (Singel 2005); and the dynamic map of conditions during the 2007 San Diego wild fires (based on individual reports) maintained by the KPBS radio station. While the sources for these maps were not crosschecked or confirmed by third parties, they provided additional data at levels of granularity and timeliness that could not be matched by other means.

Reliance on crowdsourced labor has led, however, to a return to concerns regarding the accuracy and validity of data that is not being centrally managed (Brandel 2002; Busrgener 2004) Will the maps be as good as the traditional means of mapping in disaster situations or will they contain flaws that would have been prevented by professional cartographers? While this remains a point of debate, a key benefit of peer-produced knowledge is the idea that "given enough eyeballs, all bugs are shallow" (Raymond 1999). In other words, with enough people working together, any errors by one individual can be easily corrected by another. Indeed, this crosschecking by many can be used as an argument for the superiority of peer-produced mapping over more traditional means. It has even been argued that "Internet users are faster to report earthquakes than are the seismological procedures currently in place" (Bossu et al. 2008).

Clearly the issue of quality does not lend itself to a one-size-fits-all solution. The extent to which the tensions between expert and amateur knowledge exist and are reconciled varies across both space and time. Some situations require data of the highest quality, likely only to be produced by an expert with the right set of tools and personal skills. In disaster situations, however, geographic information need only be good enough to assist recovery workers using the maps, meaning that crowdsourced information is likely to be just as helpful as that produced by more centralized means. Indeed, it can be even more useful if peer production allows for new information to be incorporated and distributed in near real time.

In addition to the division between expert and amateur knowledge production, there remains a significant gap between the liberatory potential of these technologies and their realization in practice. Although web-based mapping enables broader participation in disaster response, persistent inequality in both individual skills and access to proper tools has meant that only a relatively small and homogenous group has assisted in crowdsourced mapping (Crutcher and Zook 2009). This calls into question the oft-made claims to a Web 2.0-enabled democratic revitalization (cf. Beer and Burrows 2007).

Changes in the way that maps are accessed have also influenced their use in disaster response. With only 25.9% of the world's population having access to the Internet, but 67% having access to mobile phones (International Telecommunications Union 2009), mobile devices present a much greater possibility for access by those working in disaster response situations in developing countries. The ability of mobile devices to both create and upload new spatial data, as well as access data created by others, helps to ameliorate the limited access to full-service PCs and high-speed broadband connections.

IT applications in disaster response also allow for reciprocity between those providing information and those seeking it. Not only can experts provide assistance from nonproximate locations, but so too can locals actively seek out this help in order to gain access to otherwise inaccessible information. This is the case not only for immediate response to disasters, but also for gaining a more complete picture of potential secondary effects (Flora 2007).

Volunteered Mapping and the Haitian Crisis

"The Haiti Quake is the first disaster in which open-source, online platforms are being heavily utilized."
—Patrick Meier, director of crisis mapping at Ushahidi (Forrest 2010)

Two crucial questions that needed to be answered immediately after the earthquake hit on January 12 were: Who needs help? And where? (BBC 2010). Relief efforts had to get supplies and resources to the parts of the country most desperately in need, but it was difficult to know where to deploy resources because there was no systematic plan or data in place to help make such decisions. For decades, Haiti has been a country challenged by strife, political upheaval, and lagging economic growth, and its baseline of information infrastructure was poor. Particularly challenging to relief efforts was the fact that comprehensive databases of assets, infrastructure, population, and location were minimal. As a result, the underpinnings for an operational picture of the country before the earthquake were largely absent. Even some of the most fundamental informational needs, like detailed roadmaps and locations of critical assets, were not available.

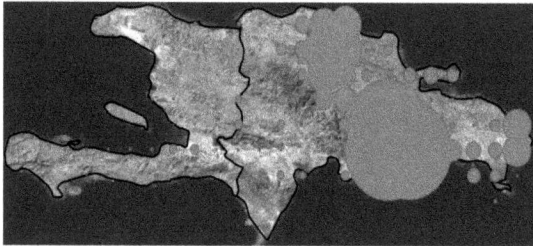

Figure 1: Number of User-Generated Placemarks Indexed by Google Maps, November 2009
Source: Author's analysis; the size of the symbol indicates the total number of user-generated placemarks. Map generated for this paper.

A compelling example of the relative lack of geo-coded information in Haiti is illustrated in Figure 1, which shows the number of user-generated placemarks (Graham and Zook 2010) on the island of Hispaniola. As can be seen, the Dominican Republic (to the east) has a much more densely populated collection of user-generated data than does Haiti (on the western portion of the island), indicating the vast disparity in available user-generated information.

Immediate Responses to the Challenges

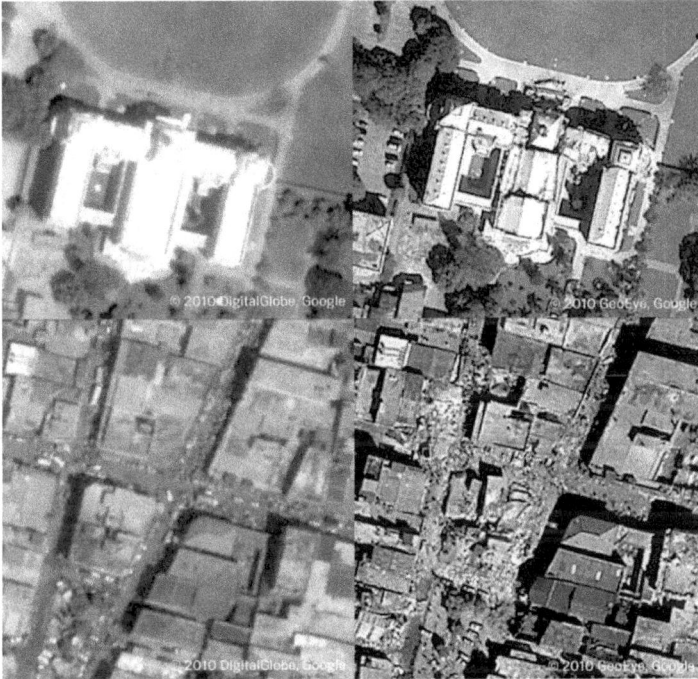

Figure 2: Before and After Satellite Images in Haiti
Source: Google (2010). Screenshot of Google website, allowed use.

Due to the dearth of available high-quality geo-information, Google, DigitalGlobe, and GeoEye worked together to get high-quality satellite imagery of post-earthquake Haiti collected, processed, and made freely available within 24 hours of the disaster (see Figure 2). This move undoubtedly helped with the coordination of emergency relief and aid services in Haiti.

Still, the lack of information complicated rescue and recovery efforts in the first days after the quake. Typical informational databases are built up over many years through GISs requiring a cadre of trained professionals to operate and maintain. However, in the Haitian crisis, much of this critical geographic information needed to build up from scratch and much of the data that was available needed to be updated based on landscape change resulting from the disaster. The years typically required to create such detailed databases now had to be accomplished in a matter of days. Even further complicating the situation was the need to identify those in need, in a country with already poor information infrastructure that had been severely damaged in the quake.

In response to this need, a rather unexpected solution appeared: volunteer community efforts matching simple web-based tools with nonprofessional data contributors. People and organizations around the world realized that they did not have to be physically present in Haiti to provide meaningful assistance to those who were. Information about opportunities to contribute spread quickly through a variety of online outlets, including blogs, emails, tweets, and status updates (see Figure 3).

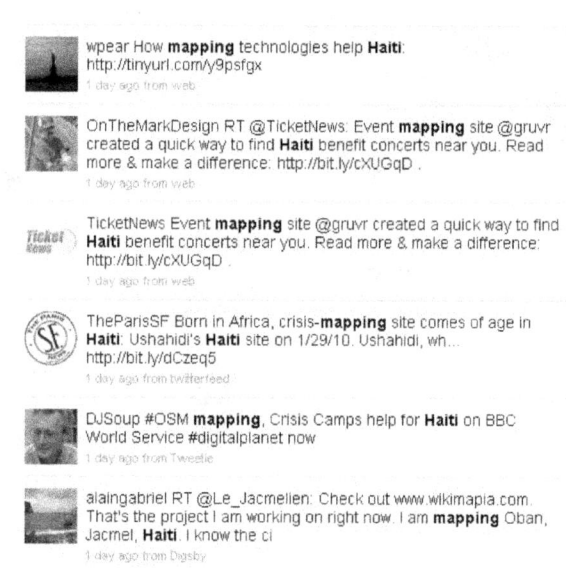

wpear How **mapping** technologies help **Haiti**:
http://tinyurl.com/y9psfgx
1 day ago from web

OnTheMarkDesign RT @TicketNews: Event **mapping** site @gruvr created a quick way to find **Haiti** benefit concerts near you. Read more & make a difference: http://bit.ly/cXUGqD .
1 day ago from web

TicketNews Event **mapping** site @gruvr created a quick way to find **Haiti** benefit concerts near you. Read more & make a difference: http://bit.ly/cXUGqD .
1 day ago from web

TheParisSF Born in Africa, crisis-**mapping** site comes of age in **Haiti**: Ushahidi's **Haiti** site on 1/29/10. Ushahidi, wh...
http://bit.ly/dCzeq5
1 day ago from twitterfeed

DJSoup #OSM **mapping**, Crisis Camps help for **Haiti** on BBC World Service #digitalplanet now
1 day ago from Tweetie

alaingabriel RT @Le_Jacmelien: Check out www.wikimapia.com. That's the project I am working on right now. I am **mapping** Oban, Jacmel, **Haiti**. I know the ci
1 day ago from Digsby

Figure 3: A Twitter Feed on February 4, 2010
Source: Twitter. Screenshot of Twitter website, allowed use.

As this example highlights, a structure and social network was in place to mobilize the tech community to support disaster relief efforts when the earthquake struck in January 2010. Projects and services such as CrisisCamp Haiti, OpenStreetMap (OSM), Ushahidi, and GeoCommons already had communities of contributors, tools, and data that could provide immediate ad hoc geographic information and situational awareness for Haiti. More importantly, their network of users and data collection tools could quickly build the needed data infrastructure for Haiti, creating an operational picture of their new reality.

CrisisCamp Haiti

CrisisCommons was formed in 2009 as a federation of citizens, NGOs, government stakeholders, and private enterprise, with the goal of better coordinating volunteer technology support during disasters. The group drew strongly from the technology community worldwide and its meetings became known as CrisisCamps. The response to the Haitian earthquake was the first widespread deployment of CrisisCommons' collective capabilities. Just four days after the earthquake struck Haiti, volunteers in Silicon Valley and Los Angeles, California, Washington, DC, New York City, and Boulder, Colorado, came together in CrisisCamps in order to begin collaborating on a variety of technology. Within another week, CrisisCamps had spread to 20 cities across the world, although the vast majority were located in the United States. Using a variety of social media tools, these groups collaborated on numerous projects meant to make the recovery effort in Haiti easier through the application of technologies.

It was clear from the start that any online mapping tools for Haiti had to account for the fact that Haitians had largely been disconnected from their already minimal connection to the Internet. This meant that delivery of the appropriate technologies required the bundling of various web components in order for their application in Haiti to work. CrisisCommons and the World Bank initiated an effort to provide vast amounts of data and tools, created by volunteers, directly to the

Haitian government. The goal was to provide simple data collection and mapping tools with a solid set of baseline data that could be built upon, such as World Bank aerial imagery, OpenStreetMap (OSM) road data, validated medical facility information, demographics, and other core operational information. These tools included an offline Haiti map browser that could run with just a hard drive or USB stick. The portable hard drives also included Delta State University's MGRS Atlases for printing map books and map images that can be viewed using Garmin handheld GPS units.

Some tools, such as We Have We Need and HaitiVoiceNeeds, were conceived of and developed by CrisisCamp volunteers specifically for application in Haiti. Although they represent just a small number of the projects worked on by the many CrisisCamps, both tools are designed to make communication between distant individuals and groups more efficient. Whether that communication is in the form of an offer or request for supplies, or a translated voice message to be sent to aid agencies, these tools have attempted to bridge the gap between those on the ground in Haiti and those who are far away, but eager to help. Although these tools have significant potential to assist aid workers, the amount of content on these sites remains relatively minimal, suggesting a limited adoption. Whether this lack of adoption is due to a lack of awareness about their benefits or an issue with the tool itself remains to be studied; however, it is clearly an issue with respect to preparation for potential disasters in the future.

In addition to their original technological contributions, Crisis-Camps also worked to provide assistance using preexisting open-source infrastructures. Spanning multiple tools, such as Akvo and Sahana, the concentrated efforts by CrisisCamp volunteers to contribute were perhaps most visible with respect to the development of OpenStreetMap (OSM) information in Haiti's urban areas. These linkages to other ongoing projects are, in many ways, mirrored by CrisisCommons' connections with the aid agencies that it seeks to support. A post on the CrisisCommons blog summarizes their work:

Working closely with the United Nations, the World Bank, and other groups providing aid, Crisis Camps everywhere have used the internet to create a powerful community with a positive purpose. Using every sort of collaborative and social media tool (open source projects, shared workspaces, Wikis, blogs, Skype, chat, twitter, facebook, etc.) *this group has pioneered a new kind of aid organization,* working hard to provide tools and information vital [to] the mission of helping Haiti recover. (CrisisCommons 2010, emphasis added)

Here the juxtaposition of a new, pioneering organization with that of the UN, World Bank, and any number of other traditional, hierarchical aid organizations is telling of the interdependencies between the two. Because of the distance and nature of assistance (technical and logistics), CrisisCommons relies upon the complementary work of on-the-ground aid agencies helping with the physical reconstruction of affected areas. At the same time, however, these relationships are much more complex, as aid agencies are growing more dependent on the skills of crowdsourced volunteers, whether they participate independently or through CrisisCamps.

OpenStreetMap

OpenStreetMap (OSM) volunteers from around the world downloaded satellite images (some already freely available and some donated by Yahoo and Google) in order to trace and record the outlines of streets, buildings, and other places of interest. These traces were uploaded into the OSM database and complemented by the work of on-the-ground volunteers in Haiti who, using portable GPS devices, were able to upload additional information (Keegan 2010). In the few weeks after the disaster, there had been nearly 10,000 edits to the Port-au-Prince region and its immediate surroundings within OpenStreetMap by hundreds of people located worldwide (Keegan 2010) (Figure 4).

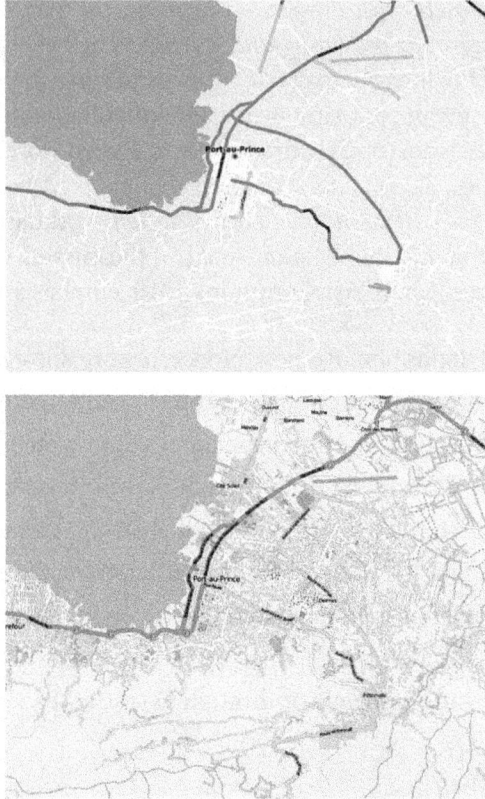

Figure 4: OpenStreetMap Before and After the Earthquake
Source: Maron (2010). Screenshot of Brainoff website, allowed use.

One important issue that came to light during the efforts to improve user-generated map coverage of Haiti was the duplication of efforts and barriers to combining data sets generated within different software packages. This issue is best illustrated via the lack of compatibility between OpenStreetMap (OSM) and another leading means for crowdsourced street maps, Google's Map Maker. Map Maker is a tool that, like OpenStreetMap, allows users to draw roads and map out areas poorly served by publicly available maps. Following the earthquake people utilized both services and started to trace out roads, hospitals, and other sites of interest. Unfortunately, due to licensing issues (OpenStreetMap issues all map data using a Creative Commons license, but Google retains the intellectual property of all information created using Map Maker), data is not portable between the two systems and efforts were undoubtedly duplicated. More importantly, this incompatibility resulted in maps with varying degrees of coverage, depending upon the location within Haiti. Figure 5 demonstrates that different parts of the country had varying levels of coverage in OpenStreetMap (OSM) (blue shading) and Map Maker (yellow shading) (Haklay 2010).

While the varying levels of information are not debilitating, this example illustrates the challenges that integrating crowdsourced data can pose. Not only should one be concerned about quality and ground-truthing, but issues of intellectual property and regulation can complicate such collaborative efforts. Despite these concerns, OpenStreetMap (OSM) and Map Maker did continue to provide rescue efforts with street map coverage extremely quickly. These spatial data were ultimately crucial for first responders, aid workers, and even U.S. military humanitarian efforts on the ground.

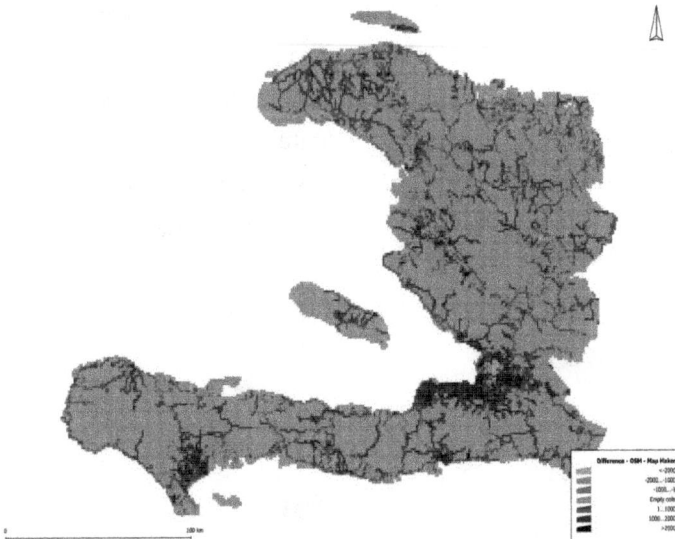

Figure 5: Difference in Coverage Between OpenStreetMap and Map Maker
Source: Haklay (2010). Screenshot of Haklay website, allowed use.

Ushahidi

A very different model of crowdsourcing was employed by the Ushahidi project. A platform with its roots in the Kenyan post-election crisis of 2008, Ushahidi users submit reports through SMS, MMS, or an online interface. Text-based reports are then geo-tagged to a particular location within an interactive map. Because of this, connections between on-the-ground events and the particular locations at which they occur are more easily discerned.

Much of this effort was set into motion by a somewhat cryptic message on Twitter posted on January 13 from Washington, DC. The message read:

> Reaching out to @FrontlineSMS users in #Haiti with hopes of establishing local SMS gateway for http://haiti.ushahidi.com

The message, written by Josh Nesbit, was an attempt to set up an emergency mobile short code for Haiti that would allow people to report various incidents via SMS. Volunteers translated messages from Creole, geo-tagged, and then placed them onto a map so that aid agencies could determine how best to employ their limited resources (see Figure 6 for an example) (BBC 2010). The U.S. State Department further assisted with the geo-location of some messages so that more reliable information could be routed to the Red Cross and U.S. Coast Guard (Knowles 2010).

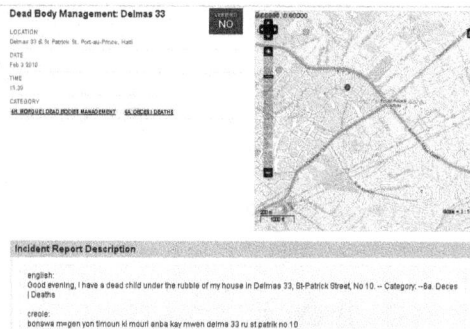

Figure 6: Report of a Dead Body on Ushahidi.com
Source: Ushahidi. Screenshot of Ushahidi website, allowed use.

It should be pointed out that the Ushahidi framework also allowed web-based and email submissions. Volunteers for Ushahidi likewise monitored all posts using the #Haiti hashtag on Twitter, and then entered the various calls for help and assistance into their publically searchable database. However, it was the ability for large amounts of local, on-the-ground knowledge to be submitted via cheap mobile devices and then systematized and shared online that distinguished Ushahidi from other projects that rely solely on the Internet as a means of user input and distribution. By allowing submissions through SMS, the system had a broad reach among the general population (only 11% of Haitians have access to the Internet compared to about a third that have access to mobile phones) (Internet World Stats 2009; Sutter 2010).

The Ushahidi project was reportedly able to make a significant impact on the relief efforts. By geo-locating urgent messages like "I'm buried under the rubble, but I'm still alive," and simply publishing relatively less immediately actionable messages such as "our community has run out of water," the project could direct people to locations in which relief actions were needed. Key to the usefulness of Ushahidi was the ability to connect short statements about problems and needs with geographic coordinates. These coordinates were then used by relief workers to find individuals and communities in need. One U.S. Marine Corps officer involved in the relief effort went so far as to state that "I cannot overemphasize to you what the work of the Ushahidi/Haiti has provided. It is saving lives every day" (Ramirez 2010).

GeoCommons

One of the challenges in the surge of VGI was ensuring that information was discoverable, interoperable, and could be repurposed across the wide variety of stakeholders involved in relief efforts. The GeoCommons project helped to achieve these objectives in the relief efforts, providing both an online and offline platform for data aggregation, dissemination, mapping, and analysis. Prior to the disaster there were less than two dozen Haiti-specific data sets and feeds in the GeoCommons project repository. Within weeks there were over 350 data sets and feeds from a multitude of sources. Data came not only from volunteers, but also from official agencies. Crowdsourcing is not limited to amateurs, and the GeoCommons project illustrated how institutions can crowdsource their internal data to facilitate better data sharing and collaboration. It is because of this that the term "volunteered geographic information" fails to fully describe the changes occurring in the creation and provision of geographic information. Crowdsourcing is about more than volunteers and amateurs. It is about creating fluidity in data sharing and collaboration by breaking down barriers in access to technology and participation through the web, open standards, and simplified interfaces. This impacts both individuals and organizations—both professionals and amateurs.

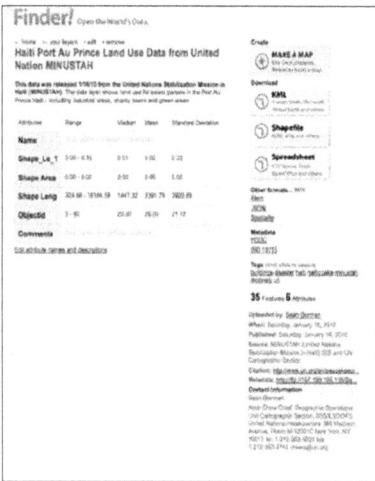

In Haiti, the GeoCommons tools not only enabled data aggregation and dissemination, but they also provided a resource for collecting metadata. Contributors could annotate the pedigree, currency, and veracity of data. An example of metadata page is provided in Figure 7.

Figure 7: Example of GeoCommons Metadata

Source: GeoCommons. Screenshot of GeoCommons website, allowed use.

This allowed data provenance to be established for the wide variety of disparate information being collected from official and unofficial sources. The tool also facilitated the repurposing of data to a variety of workflows on the ground and across the web. Data could be extracted for GIS professionals through shapefiles, Google users downloaded KML, spreadsheet users downloaded .csv, and web developers pulled content out in Atom, JSON, and Spatialite. This allowed data to be usable in a variety of venues and prevented the stove piping of critical information.

In addition, users created maps combining a variety of data sources into a single view for collaboration. This allowed maps and analysis to be personalized by users on the ground to address the specific problems they needed to address without depending on outside and scarce technical support. Figure 8 illustrates an aggregation of some of the most used sources of VGI during the early Haiti relief efforts.

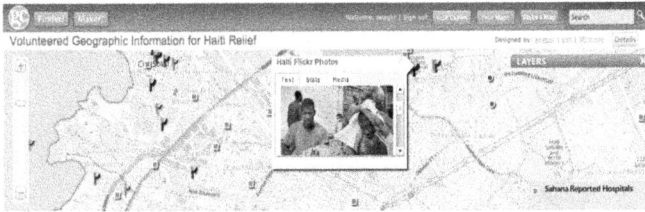

Figure 8: Example of VGI in GeoCommons
Source: GeoCommons. Screenshot of GeoCommons website, allowed use.

Historically, both data creation and mapping in the face of disaster required the skills of trained professionals. After the Haitian earthquake, relatively untrained volunteers, NGOs, and citizens were all able to create data critical to the recovery and maps that contextualized this data. There has been concern in both academia and industry about the accuracy and validity of VGI that could cause issues with accuracy and validity, possibly making it unreliable in emergency situations (Goodchild 2007). The situation and response within Haiti provide a counterexample. VGI played a critical role in emergency response in Haiti. OpenStreetMap (OSM) data was heavily used by multiple agencies and NGOs on the ground. The importance of the data is seen in feedback from emergency response workers deployed in Haiti:

> I am currently in Port Au Prince with the Fairfax County Urban Search & Rescue Team (USA-1) out of Fairfax, VA, USA. I wish there was a way that I can express to you properly how important your OSM files were to us. . . . I am spreading the word about this work to all rescue and humanitarian teams on the ground here in Haiti. Please be assured that we are using your data—I just wish we knew about this earlier. (OpenStreetMap Wiki 2010)

Data was used by on-the-ground emergency response workers as well as coordinating agencies. For instance, the U.S. Southern Command used VGI in their role coordinating disaster response for the Department of Defense. Figure 9 shows GeoCommons data and maps where VGI and official source data were fused to serve as a common operating picture for the U.S. Department of Defense Southern Command through their All Partners Access Network, which served as the collaboration point for U.S. government agencies responding to the crisis.

Figure 9: Example of GeoCommons Collaborative Mapping
Source: GeoCommons. Screenshot of GeoCommons website, allowed use.

VGI and crowdsourced disaster response played an integral role in Haiti relief efforts. It is a role, though, that complements the traditional sources of geospatial information. The largest impacts seen in Haiti were the fusion of the two sources. This combination has incredible value—providing baselines, context, and temporal adaptability to create a malleable abstract that can be molded to solve a myriad of disparate challenges.

Lessons Learned from the Haitian Earthquake Crisis

This review of efforts during the response to the Haitian earthquake highlights how people from around the world can come together (via structures like CrisisCommons) to provide assistance in times of disaster.

The first observation is that the crisis clearly resulted in a much greater availability of geo-coded data about Haiti. One can see this in the quality of aerial imagery (Figure 2), the availability of user-generated street network data (Figure 4), and the increase in data sets available via outlets like GeoCommons. A particularly striking look at the growth of crowdsourced information is provided in Figure 10, which shows the relative growth of user-generated placemarks in both Haiti and the Dominican Republic. In the brief interval between these two snapshots in time, Haiti experienced considerably more growth than the Dominican Republic, almost certainly related to the earthquake and subsequent disaster response.

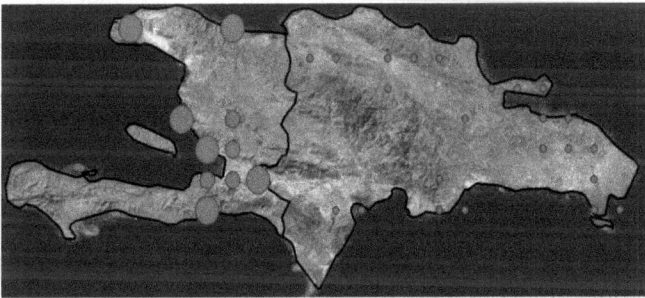

Figure 10: Change in the Number of User-Generated Placemarks Indexed by Google Maps between November 2009 and February 2010
Source: Author's analysis; the size of the symbol indicates the percentage change in usergenerated placemarks. Map generated for this paper

This increased availability of data was a function of volunteered labor using a variety of web applications. While this can produce duplication of efforts (e.g., the same streets digitized several times), this is greatly tempered by the speed at which these data sets can be produced through this decentralized structure. Moreover, duplication is not necessarily a bad thing as it can provide multiple avenues to access information. It can, however, make interpretation of a situation more complicated as multiple sources can provide conflicting versions of the built and natural environments. Furthermore, as the issues between OpenStreetMap (OSM) and Google Map Maker illustrate, nontechnical issues such as licensing can greatly complicate the combining of data sets.

These issues highlight the key role of aggregation of crowdsourced data within disaster response. Otherwise data cannot be leveraged or combined with other data sets to provide the maximum benefit for relief efforts. While typically this kind of aggregation has been provided by a government or similar organization, the Haitian crisis shows that more userdriven means of aggregation have also become viable strategies. Both Ushahidi and GeoCommons worked to aggregate data coming from multiple sources (including individual SMS messages) so that rescue teams could focus time and energy on their response rather than sorting through data.

This aggregation function (particularly the use of text messaging as an input) also highlights the importance of providing multiple channels by which data can be shared. As IT is a vulnerable and, in many cases, sparse infrastructure, disasters can destroy the capabilities (particularly Internet connections) within the affected region. Ushahidi's use of SMS highlights the benefits that come from a multi-platform approach. However, simply because a platform or service is made available does not guarantee that it will be used extensively. Such a statement should not be seen as an argument against the creation and deployment of such services, but rather an emphasis on the need to experiment widely and adapt efforts based on response and use.

Even inhabitants of a disaster zone who have access to IT (a very small percentage in the case of Haiti) may not be tied to the networks in which technology (such as Ushahidi's SMS reporting system) is made known. Accessing those most in need is a perennial challenge within economic and crisis programming, and crowdsourcing is not immune from this issue. Disasters may hit indiscriminately, but well-trod paths of economic and social standing help shape one's experience in the postdisaster world, including one's participation and access, or lack thereof, to a range of IT-driven resources (Crutcher and Zook 2009).

For example, Figure 11 shows the distribution of user-generated placemarks that make reference to the term earthquake in the Port-au-Prince region. Like other cities around the world, Port-au-Prince exhibits a pattern of clusters and empty spaces within the city (Zook 2010). However, the exact same search using a range of Haitian Creole words such as "tranblemanntè" (earthquake) or the terms for water, home, die, and hospital revealed no user-generated placemarks while searches on the English words revealed similar patterns of points to Figure 9.

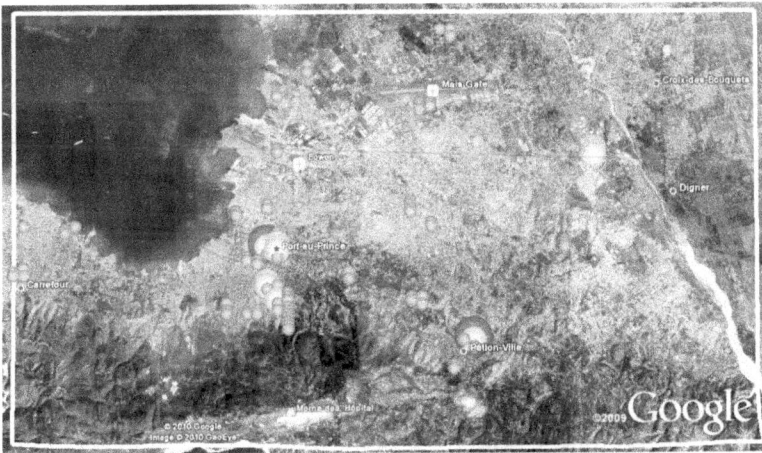

Figure 11: Number of User-Generated Placemarks Containing the Term "Earthquake," March 2010
Source: Author's analysis. Map generated for this paper.

It is therefore crucial to always recognize that user-generated content will provide only selective representations of any issue. While these representations may be highly useful to aid workers, it should not be forgotten that there will always be people and communities that are left off the map. Medical and health workers should therefore always be aware of the geographical inequalities in any crowdsourced data in order to ensure that the technologically disconnected are not denied crucial services that they may need.

Despite popular claims to the contrary, distance is not dead and the collective effort towards web-based mapping from individuals from around the world cannot change the material reality on the ground, no matter how much we wish they could. At the most basic level, the success of any disaster response depends on extremely physical factors, e.g., digging people out of the rubble, bringing in food, water, and shelter.

However, this review has also shown that crowdsourcing information and mapping services can greatly enhance the logistical systems upon which relief efforts are ultimately grounded. After all, conditions on the ground are often chaotic with multiple and conflicting inputs about priorities. The ability to aggregate, evaluate, and plan via logistical back support is a fundamental part of any response. And as the case of Haiti has shown, crowdsourcing can play a key role in these logistics.

REFERENCES

Alexander, David. 1991. "Information Technology in Real-Time for Monitoring and Managing Natural Disasters." *Progress in Physical Geography* 15 (3): 238-260.

BBC. 2010. "Crowd Sourced SMS Texts Aid Haiti Crisis." *On Click*, http://news.bbc.co.uk/2/hi/programmes/click_online/8486983.stm.

Beer, David, and Roger Burrows. 2007. "Sociology and, of and in Web 2.0: Some Initial Considerations." *Sociological Research Online* 12 (5). http://www.socresonline.org.uk/12/5/17.html.

Bossu, Remy, Gilles Mazet-Roux, Vincent Douet, Sergio Rives, Sylvie Marin, and Michael Aupetit. 2008. "Internet Users as Seismic Sensors for Improved Earthquake Response." *EOS, Transactions, American Geophysical Union* 89 (25): 225-226.

Brandel, Mary. 2002. "IT on a Mission at the American Red Cross." *Computerworld* 36 (31): 43.

Budhathoki, Nama Raj, Bertram Bruce, and Zorica Nedovic-Budic. 2008. "Reconceptualizing the Role of the User of Spatial Data Infrastructure." *GeoJournal* 72 (3-4): 149-160.

Busrgener, Eric. 2004. "Assessing the Foundation of Long Distance Disaster Recovery." *Computer Technology Review* 24 (5): 24-25.

Comfort, Louise. 1993. "Integrating Information Technology into International Crisis Management and Policy." *Journal of Contingencies and Crisis Management* 1 (1): 15-26.

CrisisCommons. 2010. "CrisisCamps Haiti—One Month Later." *CrisisCommons Blog*. February 13. http://haiti.crisiscommons.org/2010/02/crisiscamps-haiti-one-month-later/.

Crutcher, Michael, and Matthew Zook. 2009. "Placemarks and Waterlines: Racialized Cyberscapes in Post Katrina Google Earth." *GeoForum* 40 (4): 523-534.

Fischer, Henry. 1998. "The Role of the New Information Technologies in Emergency Mitigation, Planning, Response and Recovery." *Disaster Prevention and Management* 7 (1): 28-37.

Fischer, Henry. 1999. "Using Cyberspace to Enhance Disaster Mitigation, Planning and Response: Opportunities and Limitations." *Australian Journal of Emergency Management* 14 (3):60-64. http://www.ema.gov.au/5virtuallibrary/pdfs/vol14no3/fischer.pdf.

Flora, Brad. 2007. "Google Earth Impact: Saving Science Dollars and Illuminating Geo-Science." *EContent* 30 (3): 12-13.

Forrest, Brady. 2010. "Technology Saves Lives in Haiti." Forbes.com. http://www.forbes.com/2010/02/01/text-messages-maps-technologybreakthroughs-haiti_2.html.

Goodchild, Michael. 2007. "Citizens As Sensors: The World of Volunteered Geography." *GeoJournal* 69 (4): 211-221.

Google. 2010. "Haiti Imagery Layer Now Available." *Google Lat Long Blog*. January 13. http://google-latlong.blogspot.com/2010/01/haitiimagery-layer-now-available.html.

Graham, Mark. 2010a. "Cloud Collaboration: Peer-Production and the Engineering of Cyberspace." In Engineering Earth, ed. S. Brunn. New York: Springer, in press.

Graham, Mark. 2010b. "Neogeography and the Palimpsests of Place: Web 2.0 and the Construction of a Virtual Earth." *Tijdschrift voor Economische en Sociale Geografie*, Forthcoming.

Graham, Mark, and Matthew Zook. 2010. "Visualizing the Global Cyberscape: Mapping User Generated Placemarks." Unpublished paper currently under review at *Journal of Urban Technology.*

Grossman, Lev. 2006. "Time's Person of the Year: You." *Time*, December 13.

Gruntfest, Eve, and Marc Weber. 1998. "Internet and Emergency Management: Prospects for the Future." *International Journal of Mass Emergencies and Disasters* 16 (1): 55-72

Haklay, Muki. 2010. "Haiti—How Can VGI Help? Comparison of OpenStreetMap and Google Map Maker." Po Ve Sham—Muki

Haklay's personal blog. January 18. http://povesham.wordpress.com/2010/01/18/haiti-how-can-vgi-helpcomparison-of-openstreetmap-and-google-map-maker/.

Haklay, Muki, and Patrick Weber. 2008. "OpenStreetMap: User-Generated Street Maps." *IEEE Pervasive Computing 7* (4): 12-18.

Harvey, David. 2005. *A Brief History of Neoliberalism.* Oxford: Oxford University Press.

Holohan, Anne, and Anurag Garg. 2005. "Collaboration Online: The Example of Distributed Computing." *Journal of Computer Mediated Communications* 10 (4).

International Telecommunications Union. 2009. *ITU World Telecommunications/ICT Indicators Database.*

Internet World Stats. 2009. "Internet Usage Statistics." http://www.internetworldstats.com/stats.htm (accessed April 20, 2009).

Karimi, Faezeh and Danny C.C. Poo. 2009. "Personal and External Determinants of Medical Bloggers' Knowledge Sharing Behavior." Paper read at Proceedings of the Annual Meeting of the American Society for Information Science and Technology, at Vancouver, Canada.

Keegan, Victor. 2010. "Meet the Wikipedia of the Mapping World." *Guardian Unlimited.* http://www.guardian.co.uk/technology/2010/feb/04/mapping-opensource-victor-keegan.

Knowles, David. 2010. "Twitter Message Sparks Big Rescue Effort." *AOL News.* January 31. http://www.aolnews.com/tech/article/twittermessage-sparks-big-rescue-effort-in-haiti/19337648.

Kollock, Peter. 1999. "The Economies of Online Cooperation: Gifts and Public Goods in Cyberspace." *In Communities in Cyberspace,* eds. M.A. Smith, and P. Kollock. London: Routledge, 219-240.

Lakhani, Karim, and Eric von Hippel. 2003. "How Open Source Software Works: 'Free' User-to-User Assistance." *Research Policy* 32: 923-943.

Maron, Mikel. 2010. "Haiti OpenStreetMap Response". *BrainOff.* http://brainoff.com/weblog/2010/01/14/1518.

OpenStreetMap Wiki. 2010. "Talk Wiki Project Haiti." http://wiki.openstreetmap.org/wiki/Talk:WikiProject_Haiti.

Perkins, Chris, and Martin Dodge. 2008. "The Potential of User-Generated Cartography: A Case Study of the OpenStreetMap Project and Mapchester Mapping Party." *North West Geography* 8 (1): 19-32.

Preece, Jennifer, and Ben Shneiderman. 2009. "The Reader-to-Leader Framework: Motivating Technology-Mediated Social Participation." *AIS Transactions on Human-Computer Interaction* 1 (1): 13-32.

Quarantelli, E.L. 1997. "Problematical Aspects of the Information Communication Revolution for Disaster Planning and Research: Ten Nontechnical Issues and Questions." *Disaster Prevention and Management* 6 (2): 94-106.

Ramirez, Jessica. 2010. "'Ushahidi' Technology Saves Lives in Haiti and Chile." *Newsweek* blog, May 13. http://blog.newsweek.com/blogs/techtonicshifts/archive/2010/03/03/ushahidi-technology-saves-lives-in-haiti-and-chile.aspx.

Raymond, Eric. 1999. *The Cathedral and the Bazaar: Musings on Linux and Open Source by an Accidental Revolutionary.* Sebastapol, CA: O'Reilly Media.

Rodrigue, Christine. 2001. "Impact of Internet Media in Risk Debates: The Controversies Over the Cassini-Huygens Mission and the Anaheim Hills, California, Landslide." The Australian Journal of Emergency Management 16 (1): 53-61.

Rodriguez, Havidan, Walter Diaz, Jenniffer Santos, and Benigno Aguirre. 2007. "Communicating Risk and Uncertainty: Science, Technology and Disaster at the Crossroads." In Handbook of Disaster Research, eds. H. Rodriguez, E.L. Quarantelli, and R. Dynes. Berlin: Springer, 476-488.

Singel, Ryan. 2005. "A Disaster Map 'Wiki' Is Born." Wired, September 2. http://www.wired.com/software/coolapps/news/2005/09/68743.

Stephenson, Robin, and Peter Anderson. 1997. "Disasters and the Information Technology Revolution." Disasters 21 (4): 305-334.

Sui, Daniel. 2008. "The Wikification of GIS and Its Consequences: Or Angelina Jolie's New Tattoo and the Future of GIS." Computers, Environment and Urban Systems 32 (1): 1-5.

Sutter, John. 2010. "Low-Tech Radios Connect Some Haitians." CNN Online. http://www.cnn.com/2010/TECH/01/20/haiti.amateur.radio/index.ht ml.

Townsend, Anthony, and Mitchell Moss. 2005. "Telecommunication Infrastructure in Disasters: Preparing Cities for Crisis Communication." Center for Catastrophe Preparedness and Response, Robert F. Wagner Graduate School of Public Service, New York University. April 2005. http://www.nyu.edu/ccpr/pubs/NYU-DisasterCommunications1-Final.pdf.

Wohltman, Sean. 2010. "Haitian Earthquake Emphasizes Danger of a Split Geo Community." http://geosquan.blogspot.com/2010/01/haitianearthquake-emphasizes-danger-of.html (accessed February 4, 2010).

Zook, Matthew. 2010. "Metro Cyberscapes from Around the World." http://www.floatingsheep.org/2010/02/metro-cyberscapes-fromaround-world.html.

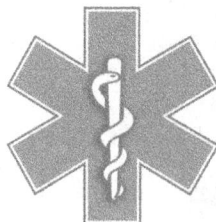

DOD AND NGOS IN HAITI—
A SUCCESSFUL PARTNERSHIP

Terbush James, *US Navy*
Miguel Cubano, *US Army*

A HISTORY OF WORKING WITH NGOS

For U.S. Southern Command, Operation Unified Response (2010 Haiti Earthquake) was not the first time the command had worked with NGOs. The linchpin of our NGO engagement strategy was the Partnering Directorate's non-governmental organization (NGO) and Business Engagement Division. This Directorate has many long-standing relationships and MOUs previously established with NGOs that operate routinely in the U.S. Southern Command Area of Responsibility (AOR). One of the major participants, Project HOPE, had worked with the U.S. Navy on many previous missions, including Operation Unified Assistance, the 2004 tsunami relief mission, and other large humanitarian disaster relief operations. The U.S. Navy's previous history with Project HOPE has served as a conduit for them to become a key partner in the execution of OPERATION CONTINUING PROMISE, the U.S. Southern Command's annual medical humanitarian relief deployment to the Caribbean Basin, Central America, and South America. The U.S. Southern Command's pre-existing relationships with the University of Miami's (Project Medishare) and Partners in Health/Haiti (Dr Paul Farmer) facilitated the sharing of information and the collaborative nature of the response. These trusted habitual partnerships made it easier to deploy together in a real-world disaster response mission.

At the time of the Earthquake disaster, there were more than 300 NGOs registered and working in Haiti. Within weeks of the catastrophe, according to the United Nations estimates, the number of NGOs reached more than 1,000. The importance of NGOs' key role in the relief efforts cannot be overstated. Not only were NGOs on the ground at the very early stages of the disaster, but more importantly they became the core element that will continue to build and sustain (in collaboration with the government of Haiti) a new and prosperous future. The evolution of DOD's relationship with NGOs is the direct result of both parties realizing the benefits of working together. Stability Operations, Humanitarian Civil Affairs as well as Humanitarian Assistance and Foreign Disaster Response (HA/FDR) operations require a significant initial influx of deployed military forces. However, such operations also require significant NGO participation, which sets the conditions for lasting peace and stability in affected countries. NGOs' long-term focus and humanitarian objectives make them a natural DoD partner for future civil–military operations.

In January 2010, the Haitian capital city of Port au Prince had the activity and energy of a country that was making a comeback from an extremely active 2008 hurricane season. Former President Bill Clinton had taken an enormous interest in Haiti's recovery and development; he had put the full weight of the Clinton Foundation behind his efforts. Hundreds of foreign investors had recently visited Haiti and were lured by the potential of a low wage workforce located only 681 miles from the largest market in the world. President Clinton's personal involvement had helped Haiti get the international community's attention and the world was finally paying attention. Savings on transportation costs alone would more than make up for Haiti's limited infrastructure and "troubled" past; Haiti was finally taking the initial steps toward becoming a feasible investment location.

On January 12, 2010, a 7.0 magnitude earthquake devastated Haiti, a country already considered to be experiencing a humanitarian emergency. United Nations estimated that more than 230,000 people were killed, 300,000 injured and 1.5 million displaced by the earthquake, (deaths and injured since revised downward). The central portion of

Port-au-Prince was significantly damaged. In addition, the airport and a dozen government buildings housing different ministries including the Ministry of Health were destroyed. The government of Haiti was practically paralyzed amidst significant chaos and uncertainty in the initial hours and days of the disaster. Almost immediately the international community, including the United States, set in motion one of the largest humanitarian disaster relief efforts in history.

The U.S. Department of State designated the U.S. Agency for International Development (USAID) as the lead federal agency for the U.S. Government response. Operation Unified Response (OUR) and the Joint Task Force Haiti (JTF-H), led by Lieutenant General Kenneth Keen, were responsible for coordinating with the United Nations, the Government of Haiti (GOH), other U.S. agencies, non-governmental organizations (NGOs) and other organizations involved in the relief efforts. One of the key assets deployed in support of this mission was the hospital ship USNS COMFORT. This over 500-bed "vessel of hope" was staffed by military personnel and NGO volunteers to provide a much-needed surgical capability to the people of Haiti.

USNS COMFORT AND NGOS IN HAITI

The hospital ship USNS COMFORT was ordered to deploy to Haiti on January 13, 2010. In approximately 72 hours the ship was on her way to Haiti to serve as a trauma hospital for earthquake victims in the Port au Prince area. Initially, the ship deployed with a crew of 850 sailors, including a medical team of 550 medical and nonmedical support staff. Within a week, however, numerous NGO personnel joined COMFORT's crew and brought it to nearly 1,200 people. NGOs provided additional critical care nursing staff, orthopedic specialists, surgical specialists, and other medical specialties. Due to ongoing contingencies in the Central Command (CENTCOM) AOR, military surgical specialists were in extremely high demand. It was extremely difficult for DoD to staff the COMFORT with the number of surgical specialists required to meet mission requirements. Because of this "gap," augmentation with NGO surgical specialists was determined to be appropriate. Within her first 40 hours on station, the COMFORT staff admitted 200 critically injured patients. Without the participation of the NGO community, COMFORT would not have been able to successfully perform 843 complex surgeries.

COORDINATION, COOPERATION, COLLABORATION (AND COMPROMISE)

In spite of all of its successes, this cooperation was not without its share of difficulties. Because of the required urgency to deploy COMFORT, she left Baltimore with only four NGO staff onboard, but not because of lack of interest on the part of NGOs. The supply of volunteers and NGO organizations willing to donate their time and expertise to the Haiti relief effort was unprecedented. U.S. Southern Command was bombarded with requests from individual volunteers as well as organizations that were seeking guidance on how to join the mission. The plan was to deploy COMFORT with the core element of approximately 500 military medical personnel, enough to be able to staff approximately 250 beds. Additional military and volunteer NGO medical staff would augment COMFORT as greater fidelity was gained on the actual needs in Port au Prince. Soon it became apparent to everyone involved that COMFORT had to be staffed so that it could operate at maximum capacity. Active duty military were initially chosen over NGO augments because they could be held on station if the mission was extended, (NGO volunteers could not be). Many civilian providers who needed to support their medical practices or other civilian jobs could only commit for a few weeks. This prioritization of military providers made some long-term NGO partners feel left out and some who were already included requested greater/longer participation. Because the length of deployment was initially undefined (and could be up to six months), a rotation of some medical staff (military or NGO) was inevitable.

The logistics required to coordinate the travel, reception, staging, and integration (RSOI) functions for NGO staff traveling from the entire United States was a daunting task. In addition, the lack of uniformity in the length of time volunteers could commit to the mission was another issue which prevented the smooth transition of the NGOs to the COMFORT. Another factor hampering the movement of volunteer staff to the COMFORT was that in the early stages of the airlift, most missions were devoted to delivering water and food supplies that were desperately needed by the Haitian population, not people. Eventually though, a total of 244 NGO and academic medical university personnel were routed through Naval Air Station Jacksonville and Naval Base Guantanamo Bay for transportation to the COMFORT.

One of the most successful areas of cooperation was between DoD and the American Red Cross (ARC). The ARC reached out to the Haitian Diasporas in: Florida, New York, and California and more than 100 Haitians residing in the United States volunteered to serve as translators onboard COMFORT during her relief efforts in Haiti. Volunteer translators were instrumental in the prompt and accurate assessment of injured Haitian patients. Translators also maintained a hotline to keep family members informed of the status of patients on board. The majority of Haitian patients also had an escort or family member who remained aboard ship until the day of discharge or transfer of the patient. Translators were invaluable to the clear understanding of medical instructions and served as a calming influence for desperate family members who wanted information about their loved ones. An unintended consequence of these additional volunteers and family members aboard COMFORT was that it reduced the maximum bed capacity significantly.

Decision making between military and NGO medical staff was coordinated through an overall NGO coordinator onboard with each of the NGOs having a lead person to represent them. Certain decisions such as the desire of some NGO staff to go ashore to continue providing medical care when COMFORT operations were complete were made by NGO's headquarters.

However, there were relatively few major decisions which were not resolved quickly with the adage of: "whatever is best for the patient."

LESSONS LEARNED AND WAY AHEAD

OPERATION UNIFIED RESPONSE has been referred to as "a model for the best disaster relief practices." The synergistic cooperation of the international community, both civilian and military, was without a doubt instrumental to the successful execution of rescue and relief efforts. Many new and innovative ideas have been presented as lessons learned from the numerous institutions involved. From the Combatant Command and Naval Component's perspective there are numerous new approaches that can be documented as lessons for other DoD entities to implement during future HA/DR operations. Among the many recommendations are: the development of a "Combined" training manual co-developed by representatives from the U.S. Military, Interagency, and NGOs. This manual would contain all relevant pertinent information required for any HA/DR stakeholder to know "what to expect" when taking part in such efforts. In addition to this manual, DoD should increase participation of NGOs and Interagency partners in exercises such as Continuing Promise and specific disaster response training. This interaction will increase each organization's comfort level with each other, allow for "role playing" in a realistic scenario, and work out idiosyncrasies and organizational procedures without the pressure of a real world event. Another recommendation was the creation of an NGO registry where NGOs could prescreen volunteers and have the ability to rapidly deploy a certain number of specialists for an agreed-upon period of time. OUR reinforced the need for increased interaction with HA/DR stakeholders. Previous interactions with non-DoD partners during OPERATION CONTINUING PROMISE enabled HA/FDR stakeholders to "hit the ground running" in support of Haiti relief operations.

Not only is increased interaction with HA/FDR stakeholders crucial to mission success, but increased educational opportunities and collective forums also enhance our collective synchronization. Instituting an academic internship program in public health and disaster medicine or staff exchanges between military and NGO/Interagency can also plant the seeds required for better understanding and smoother execution of future civil-military operations. Many of the military units that participated in OUR are conducting workshops, congresses, and conferences to discuss lessons learned in Haiti. Such forums should include: NGOs that participated in OUR, Interaction, the U.S. Department of Health and Human Services, the U.S. Agency for International Development, the U.S. Department of State, and the United Nations Office for the Coordination of Humanitarian Affairs (UNOCHA) to name a few.

On the ground in Haiti, multiple requests for assistance came from health-related NGOs and became a task for DoD. These requests typically went through USAID/Office of Foreign Disaster Assistance (OFDA) and then to the Humanitarian Assistance Coordination Center (HACC). The HACC provided additional coordination and validation of these requests and then sourced a capability to respond. Initially, a request is validated by UN Health Cluster priorities and then forwarded to the Joint Operations Tasking Center, one member of which is USAID/OFDA. OFDA in turn has the ability to form the request into the MiTaM (Mission Tasking Matrix) and after review, orders are issued by the Joint Task Force (JTF) to support the request by the NGO. In future operations and in order to speed relief supplies, the HACC process could be further resourced with knowledgeable NGO staff in the process to allow NGOs to have greater awareness of this valuable capability.

As we move along the cooperation and synchronization continuum, DoD, in coordination with the NGO community, should develop a preplanned Table of Organization (TO) to identify the size and mix of medical staff for specific types of humanitarian assistance or disaster response. This "on the shelf" TO should also include a tailored list of: equipment, logistics, and other support needs that would be best suited for a variety of HA/FDR or peacekeeping missions. The U.S. Department of Homeland Security has developed a TO for various CONUS-based contingencies. A similar approach should be taken in order to develop a TO for OCONUS-based contingencies.

Recognizing the enormous diversity of NGO expertise, the NGO community should try to standardize the wide range of competencies which volunteers bring to a given contingency. This will enable military units to have a basic understanding of the capabilities brought to bear by NGO personnel and assist in planning. Along with NGO skill standardization, the military should establish a very clear set of rules with each NGO outlining personnel qualifications and expectations for personnel participating in HA/FDR or peacekeeping operations in any part of the world. Any proposed consensus document or Memorandum of Understanding should provide: terms and conditions for deployment, redeployment, agreement related to strategic communication, cross-cultural training, and a very clear code of conduct approved by all parties. Partnership agreements based in part on past successful deployments could be created to prevent perceptions of favoritism between the military and particular NGOs. Transparency of the process is extremely important for the success of these relationships during future operations.

CONCLUSION

Civil-Military medical operations are here to stay. This interaction is not only cost-effective but also builds on the strengths of each partner. Interagency and NGO partners continue to prove their invaluable contributions to HA/FDR contingency operations. COMFORT's ability to surge and operate at full capacity was made a reality by our NGO partner's contributions to the overall effort in Haiti. Nurturing these interactions leads toward robust, stable, and long-term relationships that benefit the countries and individuals involved in disasters. A strong commitment to these relationships will likely reduce the size and duration of our military forces' commitments, freeing up additional military resources and personnel for other parts of the world and/or emerging contingencies.

REFERENCES

Beauregard, Andre. 1998. "Civil(NGO)-Military Cooperation: Lessons from Somalia, the Former, Yugoslavia, and Rwanda." *The Ploughshares Monitor* 19 (4). http://ploughshares.ca/pl_publications/civil-ngo-military-cooperation-lessons-from-somalia-the-former-yugoslavia-and-rwanda/

Bair, Andrew. 1995. "The Changing Nature of Civil-Military Operations in Peacekeeping." In *The New Peacekeeping Partnership*, ed. Alex Morrison, 66.

Conversations with VADM Michael L. Cowan regarding Military-NGO cooperation for the Future.

Pueschel, Matt. 2010. "Response to Haiti May Become Model for Disaster Relief." Health.mil, April 26, 2010.

Pollick, Sergeant Sean. 2000. "Civil-Military Cooperation: A New Tool for Peacekeepers." *Canadian Military Journal* (Autumn 2000): 57-63.

Weiss, Thomas G. 1999. *Military-Civilian Interaction: Intervening in Humanitarian Crises*. Rowman and Littlefield Publishers, New York: 11, 17.

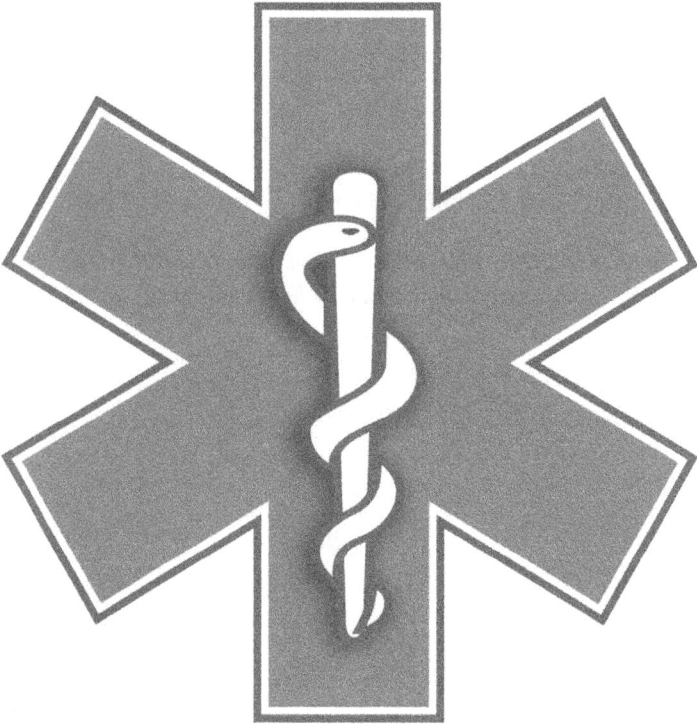

DISASTER MEDICINE:
THE NEED FOR GLOBAL ACTION

Arnauld Nicogossian, *George Mason University*
Thomas Zimmerman, *International Society of Microbial Resistance*
Otmar Kloiber, *World Medical Association*
Anatoly I. Grigoriev, Russian Academy of Sciences
Naoru Koizumi, George Mason University
Jessica Heineman-Pieper, George Mason University
Jeremy D. Mayer, GMU
Charles R. Doarn, University of Cincinnati
William Jacobs, International Society of Microbial Resistance

INTRODUCTION

The first decade of the twenty-first century was a hallmark for natural and human-made disasters. The world community continued to experience regional conflicts, terrorism, environmental degradation, death, and economic losses. Hurricanes, volcanic eruptions, earthquakes, tsunamis, floods, techno-disasters, and epidemics ravaged many countries. Whole communities were uprooted and transformed into internally displaced persons or refugees. Many suffered from extreme weather exposures, famine, and loss of basic health needs. Unfortunately the majority of the victims were poor and vulnerable population groups. Countless lives were saved and many deaths were prevented by the use of environmental monitoring and syndromic surveillance, which was made possible by the Earth remote sensing satellites and information technology. The world community responded fast with humanitarian interventions and assistance. Occasionally international aid was denied to the victims because of political differences, internal insurgency, or corruption. Despite the rapid humanitarian response and successes, economic, medical, and psychological consequences were staggering.

The 2010 economic losses alone were estimated at 222 billion USD (Swiss Re Report 2010). The mortality from natural and human-made disasters was in excess of 260,000 deaths (Swiss Re Report 2010). The Pakistan and Australian floods, the heat wave and forest fires in Russia, the devastating earthquakes in Chile, China, Haiti, and New Zealand, the BP oil rig explosion, and the subsequent Gulf of Mexico oil spill dominated the headlines around the world. Despite massive humanitarian assistance, disaster victims continue to suffer from poor living conditions, lack of sanitation, and infectious diseases. Some hard-hit disaster regions suffered epidemic ravages, such as cholera in Haiti, requiring significant public health measures (James 2010).

On January 5, 2011, U.S. Secretary of State Hillary Rodham Clinton expressed her concerns and described future challenges facing the agency's employees:

> In 2010, we faced challenges on almost every front, and our diplomacy and development efforts were put to the test. From the Middle East to the Korean peninsula and beyond, old conflicts continued to churn. Natural disasters devastated Haiti and displaced more than 20 million people in Pakistan. Around the world, millions of people—particularly women and children—suffered the ravages of war, famine, poverty and disease... In Haiti, we joined with more than 140 nations to mount one of the largest rescue and relief efforts in history. In Pakistan, we provided some 500 million USD in relief support, evacuated nearly 23,000 people, and delivered more than 16 million pounds of relief supplies. And we continued to advance global health around the world by bringing life-saving prevention, treatment, and care to more people in more places; to fight poverty, hunger, and disease; and to safeguard the rights and the roles of girls and women everywhere (Secretary Clinton 2011).

A report released by the World Bank (WB) and United Nations (UN) highlighted the cost effectiveness of prevention in reducing the death toll and economic impacts from natural disasters. This report also predicts that, by 2100, damage from extreme weather could reach 185 billion USD annually.

Disasters from climate change could add 28–68 billion USD to the overall annual costs (World Bank 2010; WMA 2009). The WB and UN report also estimates that from 1970 to 2008 natural disasters caused 3.3 million deaths.

Toward the end of 2011, the world population will pass the 7 billion mark. The number of individuals aged 65 and older will continue to grow (Hodes, Cahan, and Homer 2010). Women and children will remain vulnerable to disasters and now will be joined by the increasing aging population (McCann 2011a). The economic downturn will probably contribute to increased world disparities and some authors already warn against the "commoditization of suffering in the political economy of trauma" (James 2010).

On October 18, 2007, George W. Bush issued a Homeland Security Presidential Directive (HSPD-21) on public health and disaster medical preparedness. HSPD-21 specifically calls for developing "a mechanism to coordinate public health and medical disaster preparedness and response core curricula and training across executive departments and agencies, to ensure standardization and commonality of knowledge, procedures, and terms of reference within the Federal Government that also can be communicated to State and local government entities, as well as academia and the private sector." Following the HSPD-21 a number of studies addressing the competencies for "disaster medicine" training were published (Subbaro et al. 2008; King et al. 2010). These studies highlighted that preparedness and recovery are far from optimal and that there is a lack of evidence-based information, with the exception of a limited number of lessons learned from previous disasters to guide future medical practices and skill training. The American Board of Disaster Medicine continues to address the competencies in this new discipline and additional international effort will be required to ensure consistency in training and proper use of community resources (McCann 2011b, Nicogossian et al. 2011).

By recognizing cross-cultural commonalities and differences, the disaster medicine practice can potentially provide solutions for better public health and medical care delivery (Farmer 2005). We propose that Disaster Medicine competencies and training should also emphasize ethics (WMA 2006), international law, medical diplomacy, advocating victims' special needs, concerns and rights. Disasters will continue to happen and proper support, through a granting program, will be necessary to explore and bench mark best practices in Disaster Medicine.

REFERENCES

Farmer, Paul. 2005. *Pathologies of Power.* Berkeley, CA: University of California Press.

Hodes, Richard J., Vicky Cahan, and Megan J. Homer. 2010. "Aging Research: Translating Scientific Discovery into Clinical Intervention." *World Medical & Health Policy* 2 (4): Article 2.

James, E.C. 2010. "Ruptures, Rights and Repair: The Political Economy of Trauma in Haiti." *Social Science & Medicine* 70: 106-113.

King, R.V., C.S. North, G.L. Larkin, et al. 2010. "Attributes of Effective Disaster Responders: Focus Group Discussions with Key Emergency Response Leaders." *Disaster Medicine Public Health Preparedness* 4 (4): 332-338. HSPD-21: www.dhs.gov/xabout/laws/gc_1219263961449.shtm (accessed January 16, 2011).

McCann, D. 2011a. "A Review of Hurricane Disaster Planning for the Elderly." *World Medical & Health Policy* 3 (1): 5-30.

McCann, D. 2011b. "Developing International Standards for Disaster Preparedness and Response: How Do We Get There?" *World Medical & Health Policy* 3 (1): 1-4.

Nicogossian, A.N., et al. 2011. "The Use of U.S. Academic Institutions in Community Medical Disaster Recovery." *World Medical & Health Policy.* 3 (3): 1-12.

Secretaryclinton.wordpress.com/2011/.../secretary-of-state-hillary-clintons-memo-to-her-staff-a-busy-year-ahead-for-diplomacy/ (accessed January 30, 2011).

Subbaro, I., et al. 2008. "A Consensus-based Educational Framework and Competency Set for the Discipline of Disaster Medicine and Public Health Preparedness." *Disaster Medicine Public Health Preparedness* 2: 57-68.

Swiss Re Report. 2010. "Preliminary Estimates for 2010 from Swiss Re Sigma Show that Natural Catastrophes and Man-made Disasters caused Economic Losses of USD 222 Billion and Cost Insurers USD 36 Billion." www.swissre.com (accessed January 24, 2011).

WMA Declaration of Delhi on Health and Climate Change 2009. www.wma.net/en/30publications/10policies/c5/index.html.

WMA Statement on Medical Ethics in the Event of Disasters 2006. www.wma.net/en/30publications/10policies/d7/index.html.

World Bank. 2010. "Natural Hazards, Unnatural Disasters: The Economics of Effective Prevention." http://www.gfdrr.org/gfdrr/sites/ gfdrr.org/files/nhud/files/NHUD-Overview.pdf

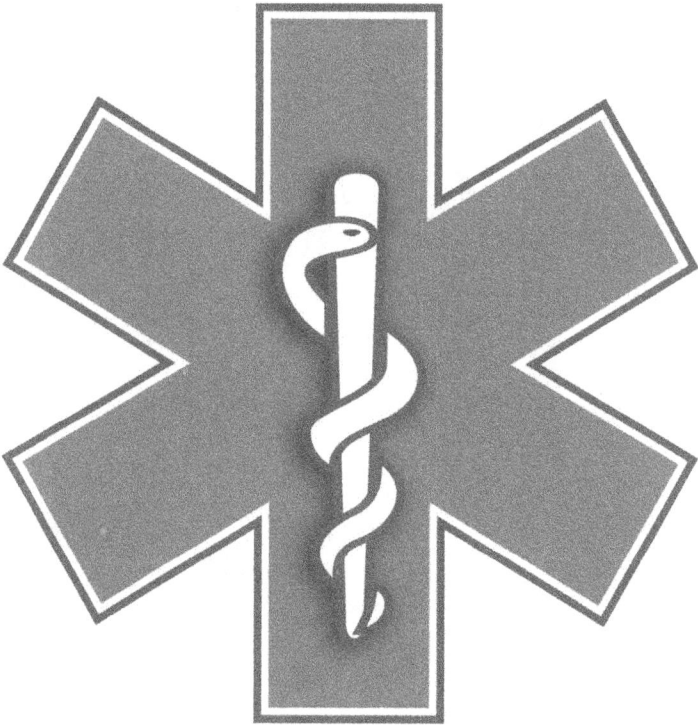

POVERTY, DISPARITIES, DISASTERS, AND GLOBAL BURDEN OF DISEASE

Arnauld Nicogossian, *George Mason University*
Otmar Kloiber, *World Medical Association*
Thomas Zimmerman, *International Society of Microbial Resistance*
Bonnie Stabile, *George Mason University*
Kevin Thomas, *Boston University, School of Medicine*
James W. Terbush, *American Academy of Disaster Medicine*
Charles R. Doarn, *University of Cincinnati*

On January 16, 2012, the United Nations (UN) released the 2011 annual Millennium Development Goals (MDG) progress report. The report finds that "significant strides towards achieving the MDGs have been made, yet reaching all the goals by the 2015 deadline remains challenging because the world's poorest are being left behind." The worsening global economy and rising energy costs have contributed to higher unemployment and increased poverty around the world. Adding to the suffering of millions, the frequency and severity of natural disasters continue to rise, affecting ever larger segments of the world population. Surpassing 2010 estimates, 2011 become another costly year due to natural disasters.

In 2011, natural disasters were responsible for more than 600 deaths in the United States and an estimated 59 billion USD in damages (FEMA 2012; NOAA 2011). The Great Eastern Japan Earthquake of March 2011 claimed 19,846 lives, and in December 2011 over 1,400 people lost their lives in tropical storms and flooding in Australia, New Zealand, the Philippines, and Thailand. Europe experienced very few disasters in 2011 with the lowest numbers killed and economic damages since 1990. Almost 45% of all disasters occurred in Asia accounting for 85% of all casualties and almost 75% of total economic damages. It is estimated that 2011 has been the costliest year ever at a staggering 380 billion USD (Samenow 2011).

Disasters are complex events which multiply environmental and health hazards in the post-recovery period (Nicogossian et al. 2011a; 2011b). Despite the efforts of the UN and developed countries, and progress to reduce health disparities, many states experiencing recurrent natural disasters continue to report poor health outcomes and inequalities (Frieden et al. 2011; Zaidi, Kamal, and Baig-Ansari 2010). In the United States, rural and vulnerable populations share a larger burden of morbidity and mortality during the recovery period following disasters (Davis et al. 2010; Fothergill and Peek 2004; Fox et al. 2010; Fussell, Sastry, and VanLandingham 2010; Toldson et al. 2011). A recent survey of Katrina survivors identified major differences in the rates of life expectancy, educational attainment, and incomes of African Americans and Caucasians in Louisiana (Fox et al. 2010; Toldson et al. 2011).

Disasters tend to magnify health disparities. The poor and the unemployed living on the brink of socioeconomic and health collapse are resource constrained and have limited access to medical and health services within their communities. Vulnerable populations also experience a higher risk of psychological, acute, and chronic diseases following disasters. For example, neighborhood-level income inequality has been associated with depression among persons with lower income and food insecurity and can contribute to obesity (Ivers and Cullen 2011). This group may be more socially or economically marginalized and dependent on local welfare than the wealthy whose personal resources offer them more choices (Fussell et al 2010) In New Orleans, when Hurricane Katrina struck, many people with chronic health conditions, relying heavily on the public hospital system, found most of the healthcare system destroyed in the storm (Brodie et al. 2006), leaving them without expected services. Children and adolescents are particularly vulnerable to the effects of disasters. After Hurricane Katrina, 37% of children were diagnosed with clinical depression, anxiety, or behavioral disorders (Abramson et al. 2010). Following the 2010 Haiti earthquake, there was an increased incidence of trauma, injury, diarrhea, and suspected malaria in rapidly growing, crowded tent settlements, which were also lacking in sanitation, exacerbating medical problems, especially among children.

Benchmarking for long-term recovery should address individuals, businesses, communities, aid organizations, social entrepreneurs, and state, local, and federal governments. Some best practices should consider benchmarking the role of social entrepreneurs and their interactions with the affected community (Chamlee-Wright and Storr 2009). Social entrepreneurs' role after a disaster is described as "often alert to neighborhoods' needs in a way that government agencies are not. Social entrepreneurs don't just fill the gaps in needed services—they also work to galvanize the support that is essential for community resilience" (Chamlee-Wright and Storr 2009).

Both the U.S. Healthy People 2020 and the UN MDGs recognize the importance of removing disparities to improve long-term individual health outcomes and the quality of life. Recognition is an important element of preparedness, but does not necessarily result in positive and integrated action among all stakeholders. Intervention measures such as standardizing outcome measures, establishing disaster-specific registries addressing knowledge gaps, and priority funding for programs designed to remove health disparities and improve population health in the regions at risk (Davis et al. 2010), together with integrating strategic resources to minimize duplication of effort should be understood and implemented. Coordination among different stakeholders to ensure effectiveness of meeting health milestone before disaster strikes is a priority for national and international health services agencies and organizations.

Consistent and reliable disaster recovery and long-term health indicators are not always available or used (Koehlmoos 2010). Following the 2004 Indian Ocean tsunami and the 2005 Pakistan earthquake, mental health and women's health and maternal mortality, were, respectively, used as indicators of success (de Mel, McKenzie, and Woodruff 2008; Miller and Arquilla 2007). Indicators for long-term recovery should be further evaluated, standardized, and benchmarked in order to help communities and governments benchmark chronic health risks and invest in effective preparedness practices for the next disaster(s).

REFERENCES

Abramson, D.M., Y.S. Park, T. Stehling-Ariza, and I. Redlener. 2010. "Children as Bellwethers of Recovery: Dysfunctional Systems and the Effects of Parents, Households, and Neighborhoods on Serious Emotional Disturbance in Children after Hurricane Katrina." *Disaster Medicine and Public Health Preparedness*. Published online August 23, 2010. http://www.ncdp.mailman.columbia.edu/files/dmp.pdf (accessed January 10, 2012).

Brodie, M., E. Weltzien, D. Altman, R.J. Blendon, and J.M. Benson. 2006. "Experiences of Hurricane Katrina Evacuees in Houston Shelters: Implications for Future Planning." *American Journal of Public Health* 96 (8): 1402-1408.

Chamlee-Wright, E., and V.H. Storr. 2009. "Post-Disaster Recovery and Social Entrepreneurship." http://localknowledge.mercatus.org/articles/post-disaster-recovery-and-social-entrepreneurship/ (accessed January 26, 2012).

Davis, J.R., S. Wilson, A. Brock-Martin, S. Glover, and E.R. Svendsen. 2010. "The Impact of Disasters on Populations with Health and Health Care Disparities." *Disaster Medicine and Public Health Preparedness* 4 (1): 30-38.

de Mel, S., D. McKenzie, and C. Woodruff. 2008. "Mental Health Recovery and Economic Recovery After the Tsunami: High-frequency Longitudinal Evidence from Sri Lankan Small Business Owners." *Social Science & Medicine* 66 (3): 582-595.

FEMA. 2012. "Federal Disaster Declarations." www.fema.gov/disasters.fema (accessed January 31, 2012).

Fothergill, A., and L.A. Peek. 2004. "Poverty and Disaster in the United States: A Review of Recent Sociological Findings." *National Hazards* 32, 89-110.

Fox, M.H., et al. 2010. "The Psychosocial Impact of Hurricane Katrina on Persons with Disabilities and Independent Living Center Staff Living on the American Gulf Coast." *Rehabilitation Psychology* 55 (3): 231-240.

Frieden, T.R., et al. 2011. "CDC Health Disparities and Inequalities Report— United States 2011." *MMWR Supplement*; Vol. 60.

Fussell, E., N. Sastry, and M. VanLandingham. 2010. "Race, Socioeconomic Status and Return Migration to New Orleans after Hurricane Katrina." *Population and Environment* 31 (1–3): 20-42.

Ivers, L.C., and K.A. Cullen. 2011. "Food Insecurity: Special Considerations for Women." *American Journal of Clinical Nutrition* 94 (6): 1740S-1744S. Epub November 16, 2011.

Koehlmoos, T.P. 2010. "Evidence aid and the Disaster Response in Pakistan and and Haiti." *Cochrane Database Systematic Reviews*. ED000014 (accessed February 1, 2012).

Miller, A.C., and B. Arquilla. 2007. "Disasters, Women's Health, and Conservative Society: Working in Pakistan with the Turkish Red Crescent Following the South Asian Earthquake." *Prehospital Disaster Medicine* 22 (4): 269-273.

Nicogossian, A., T. Zimmerman, O. Kloiber, A.I. Grigoriev, N. Koizumi, J. Heineman-Pieper, J.D. Mayer, C.R. Doarn, and W. Jacobs. 2011a. "Disaster Medicine: The Need for Global Action." *World Medical & Health Policy* 3 (1): Article 1.

Nicogossian, A., T. Zimmerman, O. Kloiber, B. Stabile, R.C. Doarn, J.W. Terbush, and M.A. Ramirez. 2011b. "Medical and Public Health Consequences of 2001." *World Medical & Health Policy* 3 (3): Article 1.

NOAA. 2011. "A Year of Climate Extremes in the United States." www.noaanews.noaa.gov/stories2012/20120119_global_stats.html (accessed January 31, 2012).

Samenow, Jason. 2011. "Munich Re: Unprecedented Year for Natural Disasters." *The Washington Post*, July 13. http://www.washingtonpost.com/blogs/capital-weather-gang/post/munich-re-unprecedented-year-for-natural-disasters/2011/07/13/gIQAghxSCI_blog.html (accessed January 31, 2012).

Toldson, I.A., et al. 2011. "Examining the Long-term Racial Disparities in Health and Economic Conditions Among Hurricane Katrina Survivors: Policy Implications for Gulf Coast Recovery." *Journal of Black Studies* 42 (3): 360-378.

Zaidi, S., A. Kamal, and N. Baig-Ansari. 2010. "Targeting Vulnerabilities after the 2005 Earthquake: Pakistan's Livelihood Support Cash Grant Programmes." *Disasters* 34 (2): 380-401.

III.
LOGISTICAL CONSIDERATIONS IN DISASTER RESPONSE

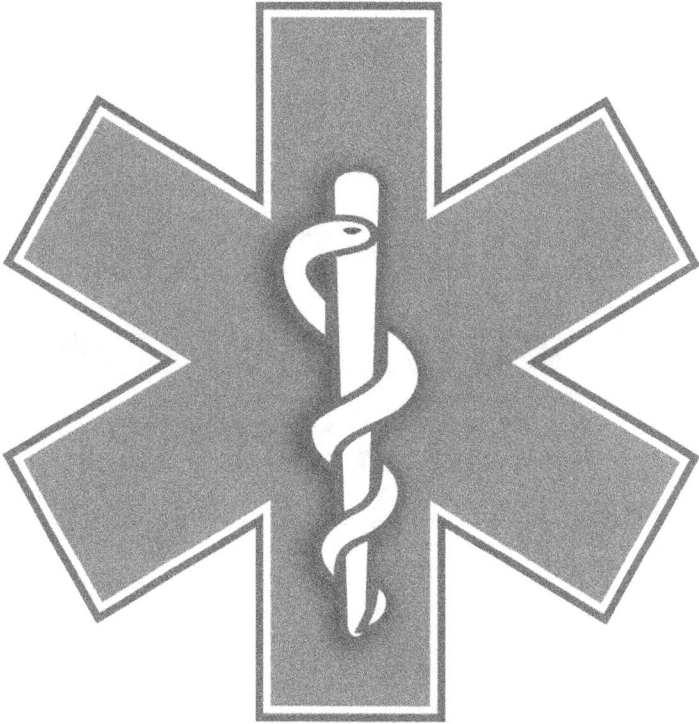

MAXIMIZING UTILITY OF A DEPLOYABLE MEDICAL TEAM FROM AN ACADEMIC MEDICAL CENTER TO A DISASTER

Christina L. Catlett, *Johns Hopkins University*
Thomas D. Kirsch, *Johns Hopkins University*
James J. Scheulen, *Johns Hopkins University*
Gai Cole, *Johns Hopkins University*
Gabor D. Kelen, *Johns Hopkins University*

INTRODUCTION

Academic medical centers (AMCs) have tremendous potential as a valuable response asset to regions affected by disasters or other healthcare crises. AMCs have a large pool of faculty and staff with a variety of clinical, administrative, logistical, and subject matter expertise, some of whom have considerable experience in disaster or humanitarian response in a variety of theaters and conditions. Furthermore, larger AMCs often have sufficient flexibility to allow staff to respond and maintain response continuity if rotation in and out of theater is required. The purpose of this article is to describe the development of a deployable medical team at the Johns Hopkins Institutions (JHI) and the operational lessons learned during its first deployment, the 2010 Haiti earthquake.

BACKGROUND

The capacity of the U.S. government, non-governmental organiza tions (NGOs), and the U.S. military to respond to disasters, particularly catastrophic events, is often limited by the number of available personnel and specific technical expertise. The pool of full-time disaster responders is very small. For example, the U.S. government's Office of Foreign Disaster Assistance (OFDA) has fewer than 300 staff and consultants to cover events around the globe and to maintain operations at its headquarters in Washington, DC, and its international regional offices (USAID 2009). These limitations compel responding agencies to seek additional personnel from external sources during major disasters. Through trained deployable disaster teams, AMCs have significant capacity and potential as a valuable response partner for NGOs and the Department of Defense (DOD) during major disasters.

LITERATURE REVIEW

There are a number of ways in which AMCs are providing disaster response assets. For example, Carolinas Medical Center in North Carolina and Hackensack University Medical Center in New Jersey have developed mobile hospitals that may be deployed to an area in crisis to provide emergency, surgical, and critical care services (Blackwell and Bosse 2007; Schunk 2009). Some AMCs work closely with NGOs to provide staffing support during times of crisis, such as the University of Miami and its work with Project Medishare in Haiti (Ginzburg et al. 2010). Six Chicago medical institutions formed a collaborative initiative known as the Chicago Medical Response which partnered with NGOs in Haiti following the earthquake to provide a sustained post-disaster response of medical providers (Babcock et al. 2010). The University of Pennsylvania collaborated with a well-established NGO to provide anesthesia and surgical services in Haiti (McCunn et al. 2010). AMCs can also be associated with, or largely staff, a Disaster Medical Assistance Team (DMAT), part of the National Disaster Medical System (NDMS) that augments the U.S. medical response capability to critical events. The University of New Mexico Health Sciences Center (Sklar et al. 2007), Mass General Hospital (Gaudette et al. 2002), and more recently the Johns Hopkins Institutions are strongly identified with respective DMATs in their state.

AMCs can also create their own unaffiliated rapidly deployable medical teams that could be requested as a local, state, tribal, federal, or DOD asset, or as a private asset by an NGO, a foreign government, or private entity (e.g., a hospital).

METHODS

In 2008, the Johns Hopkins Office of Critical Event Preparedness and Response (CEPAR) received a grant from the Health Resources and Services Administration (HRSA) to build a deployable disaster medical asset named the "Johns Hopkins Go Team." Recruitment began in 2009 and included physicians, physician extenders, nurses, technicians, respiratory and physical therapists, pharmacists, dieticians, mental health providers, logistics specialists (facility and supply managers), administrative and financial staff, safety officers, security personnel, health informatics and communications specialists, environmental engineers, epidemiologists, and disaster researchers. Based on our previous disaster experience, anticipated capabilities of the Go Team included mass casualty triage, staffing of field clinics for victims, medical support to shelters, backfill in hospitals, and public health services such as conducting surveys and providing vaccinations.

A rigorous pre-deployment educational program for the Go Team was developed using various formats to achieve core competencies (Subbarao et al. 2008). Members became certified in two Federal Emergency Management Agency (FEMA) courses: IS-700 (National Incident Management System, An Introduction) (FEMA 2011) and ICS-100 HC (Introduction to the Incident Command System for Healthcare/Hospitals) (FEMA 2010). Basic Disaster Life SupportTM (BDLS®) and Advanced Disaster Life SupportTM (ADLSTM) provided Go Team members with important skills to respond to a disaster setting (National Disaster Life Support Foundation 2007). The team completed web-based interactive, multi-media educational modules on a variety of disaster topics (Medfilms Online Inc. 2009). Team members were also offered a new course entitled "Advanced Field Provider Training," which was designed and implemented at our institution through a grant from the Centers for Disease Control (CDC, grant # 5U90TP324236-05). This four-part course is a combination of presentations on real-world disaster experiences and hands-on workshops on practical in-field skills. Finally, members were offered education in psychological first aid.

Two leadership courses were held to develop a group of core team leaders: a three-day Outward Bound Professional Program (2011) that focused on leadership skills, teamwork and team building, communication skills, deployment responsibilities, and use of specialized equipment; and a leadership development seminar that focused on communication, improvisation, and creativity in emergency situations.

RESULTS

When the earthquake struck Haiti on January 12, 2010, an estimated 230,000 were killed, and 1 million were left homeless (USAID 2010). CEPAR was tasked by JHI leadership with preparing for potential disaster assistance for the earthquake via the Go Team. We quickly realized the challenges in deploying our new team to Haiti given its original concept as a human resource asset. Inserting a team into Haiti without a formal invitation, well-defined mission, security plan, and self-sustaining supplies of food, water, shelter, and medical goods was not a responsible option and would have added additional burden to the region (Van Hoving et al. 2010). However, through adaptation of our concept of operations, strategic partnership with established response agencies, and thoughtful management of the deployed team's logistics and operations, we were able to respond effectively to this international crisis. The following summarizes key lessons learned that have been incorporated into a new concept of operations document for our deployable AMC team.

Value of Partnership with Established Response Organizations

Deploying to austere environments like the disaster in Haiti where logistics are challenging and response resources are already limited requires that teams be entirely self-sufficient for personal needs and for the equipment and supplies necessary to provide services. Healthcare providers, especially hospital-based providers, should ideally be paired with a well-established organization that has a logistical infrastructure in place (McCunn et al. 2010). Pre-trained medical teams from AMCs are an excellent adjunct to military and NGO response, particularly when our U.S. military medical providers are spread thin on multiple fronts. However, in order to make this idea operational and to prevent logistical delays, there must be well-developed MOUs that delineate specific roles and capacities, limitations of activities, and reporting structures to allow for quick deployment.

Our institution, particularly through the School of Public Health, has a long history of collaborating with international NGOs throughout the world. The first Go Team group deployed with the International Medical Corps (IMC), a respected organization with more than 25 years of international relief experience. IMC had a need for medical personnel to staff their operations at a large damaged hospital in Port-au-Prince. Their needs and defined mission were well matched with our capabilities, and their on-ground logistics, support services, and security were the resources that we sought. The John Hopkins Hospital Go Team deployed five physicians, three nurses, and one nurse practitioner with IMC to the Hopital de l'Universite d'Etat d'Haiti (University Hospital). They arrived 14 days after the earthquake to staff and manage the emergency care areas and treated traumatic injuries, wound infections, endemic infectious diseases such as tetanus and tuberculosis, and decompensation of chronic medical issues. The team, with other U.S. and Haitian physicians, worked 12–14-hour shifts to treat 400–500 patients per day over a two-week period.

We also collaborated with the DOD to provide Go Team human resources. Our geographic proximity to the Naval hospital ship USNS Comfort, berthed in Baltimore, made it a logical choice for partnership. Liaisons with the Navy had been established in 2002, and there were significant discussions regarding collaboration during Hurricane Katrina in 2005. The Navy was developing a plan to incorporate civilian support for the Haiti response. JHI developed an MOU directly with the Navy which set forth the terms of the resource sharing partnership. Two teams were deployed to the USNS Comfort under the new MOU, each for two weeks. The first team (an anesthesiologist and a nurse anesthetist) arrived three weeks after the earthquake and helped manage the large influx of patients with complex orthopedic and neurosurgical trauma. The second team, comprised of an emergency physician, two nurses, and a pediatric nurse practitioner, arrived five weeks after the disaster and provided ongoing support during the Comfort's initial demobilization efforts, including discharge planning of earthquake victims from the ship to Haitian facilities.

Flexible and Modular Team Structure

Structural flexibility in the source and expertise of personnel proved a hallmark of success for the Go Team. By design, Go Team members were recruited not only from various clinical departments but also from different hospitals within our institution. This strategy optimized our ability to respond readily to the needs of multiple missions without degrading staff at one particular hospital or department that could compromise patient care. Detailed and proactive planning for sustainable response through staggered deployment blocks prevented institutional disruption and responder fatigue over long-term responses.

Each disaster has different healthcare needs. One of the inherent values of basing a response team at an AMC is the ability to quickly vet the suitability of healthcare providers or subject matter experts needed to augment the existing team. While deployment of untrained team members is not ideal, selection of auxiliary members with previous disaster or humanitarian experience is helpful. The role of remote medical direction from non-deployed specialties and telemedicine is an option that may be explored in future deployments by the Johns Hopkins Go Team.

The Value of Training

A significant challenge in using outside personnel to meet the acute needs of a disaster response is their lack of training, knowledge, and/or experience in providing care in an austere environment (Jobe 2011). The Go Team educational program was designed to give providers (especially those with no austere environment experience) the tools and skills they would need to operate effectively in the field. For example, training in ICS and NIMS was deemed to be critical to domestic response. We learned from the Haiti disaster that further training in international in-field integration and collaboration is equally important. As a result, we are exploring additional training in the United Nations cluster system, the role of the United States Agency for International Development (USAID) in response, and an overview of other key international response agencies as critical skill sets for internationally deployed Go Team members.

Responding agencies may not request a full, large team. Rather, the needs are dictated by the mechanism of disaster and tend to be for specific types of providers. The implication of our experience is that an AMC-based response team may not need to spend time training as a large team (as DMATs do) since it is unlikely they will deploy "en masse." Efforts are better spent making sure team members are competent to operate individually or in small teams in very austere environments where there may be little in the way of support infrastructure. Just-in-time training specific to the destination environment may also play a role; for example, we have developed an educational module on operating within a military ship environment.

Pre-deployment Logistics

It is critical to understand the deployment environment and its associated health, security, and licensure issues. Prior to Haiti deployment, briefings were held to present each team's mission, educate members about the destination environment, discuss packing lists, and address any questions or concerns of deployed members. Members were also screened for suitability for deployment to Haiti; we felt that due to the severe lack of infrastructure (Kirsch and Moon 2010), members should be in reasonable physical condition and generally healthy. Appropriate immunizations were arranged, as well as prophylactic medications (e.g., anti-malarials and post-exposure prophylaxis). The AMC must take into consideration whether the institution will cover the cost of immunizations and prophylaxis (as we did), or if the volunteer must bear the cost, as travel immunizations are not covered by many insurance plans.

Chain of Command

The designation of a team leader and a deputy leader was important to in-field operations and integration with NGO leadership and Navy incident command. The team leader in all cases was the most experienced senior deployed member; two of the three leaders had received prior Go Team leadership training. The leader managed credentialing in the field and was responsible for the assignments, actions, and welfare of all members of the team. The team leader had authority to make decisions based on "facts on the ground," but was required to report daily when possible to CEPAR stateside. This combination of "agility and discipline"—working within a complex organizational structure while using adaptability and improvisation to efficiently deliver care—has been advocated by Harrald (2006) as a critical hallmark of success for disaster response. Job action sheets outlining expectations of the leader and deputy roles were developed and refined after each deployment.

Communications and Situational Awareness

Communication during this catastrophe was vital to both the in-field teams and the home institution. Once on the ground, contact between teams and with leadership at our institution proved extremely difficult. Although each team had been equipped with a satellite phone, they were felt to be more effective for outgoing calls than incoming since the team could not leave the phone on to preserve battery life. Having access to multiple modes of communication, such as sat phones, handheld radios, cell phones, and Internet (if available), increases the likelihood of successful communication. Team members should receive just-in-time training on sat phones and radios; providing the team with a solar charger may be vital in austere environments.

Post-deployment follow-up

Working in a disaster zone is inherently physically and mentally stressful, to both professional rescue personnel and volunteers (Thormar et al. 2010; Brackbill et al. 2006). Post-deployment health screening was carried out through our Travel Medicine clinic, including six-month TB testing follow-up. The physical hardships and sheer magnitude of devastation and death in Haiti compounded the psychological stress placed on volunteers who deployed. The Johns Hopkins Faculty and Staff Assistance Program (FASAP) was engaged early in the deployment process so that appropriate mental health follow-up could be implemented for all team members who responded to the disaster. FASAP faculty attended the group debriefing to speak to those deployed and followed up individually with each person.

Complexity of Human Resource (HR) Issues

The decision to deploy personnel as employees of an institution versus allowing employees to freely volunteer with an NGO or another organization is complex. Employees deploying as individual volunteers generally accept the risk of deployment and work under the legal protection of the NGO or sponsoring agency (if offered), not of their primary employer. In such situations, the employee must use personal time (vacation time or paid time off) during deployment. Institutions that decide to deploy personnel as employees of the organization, as we did with the U.S. Navy, accept the risk and responsibility for the actions and potential injuries of those employees as if they were continuing to work onsite. The decision to cover salaries, potential requirement of overtime pay for staff in certain employment positions, and coverage of malpractice, liability, and workers compensation were complex issues that required significant input and discussion with both HR and risk management.

The Cost of Deployment

Although the concept of humanitarian assistance is noble and compelling, it is an interesting challenge to make the financial argument for AMC participation in an endeavor that is not part of its core mission, and at a considerable expense for the institution. Deploying personnel in any manner carries with it some significant cost, which may include the salary of the deployed personnel and additional costs related to backfill personnel, overtime pay, malpractice and liability insurance, health insurance, travel insurance, workers compensation, travel costs, immunizations, and team gear, supplies, and equipment. Our institution was willing to assume reasonable financial responsibility in order to realize a meaningful response to the Haitian catastrophe. An AMC may be able to distribute the cost of deployment across different entities or departments within its institutions so that no single clinical department or even one hospital need bear the full financial burden.

Ongoing Team Development

Given the time and effort put into recruiting, training, and maintaining a large cadre of deployable volunteers at an AMC, it is beneficial to allow members to serve in some fashion and gather experience during non-disaster times. Because of our MOU with the Navy, we are supporting the Navy's ongoing humanitarian mission in the Caribbean and Central/South America (Operation Continuing Promise). Collaboration during non-disaster times allows AMC deployment team members to provide humanitarian assistance, gain experience in delivering healthcare to underdeveloped nations and in austere conditions, and (in our case) to become familiar with Navy customs, standard operating procedures, and mission priorities (Marklund et al. 2010). It also allows the AMC to build leadership, trust, and legitimacy within the partner organization, a cornerstone of cross-sector collaboration proposed by Bryson, Crosby, and Stone (2006).

In order to establish the Go Team as a federally recognized asset and to explore the possibility of ongoing funding to support team administration, we have registered the team as a formal Medical Reserve Corps (MRC) team. The MRC designation allows the Go Team visibility at the state and federal level as an available asset for future deployments.

CONCLUSION

Deployable medical teams from academic healthcare institutions can provide a valuable adjunct to disaster and humanitarian response. Collaboration with well-established response agencies such as NGOs or with the U.S. military can be mutually beneficial, as response organizations usually require personnel or subject matter experts, and AMCs frequently require logistical support and security in the field. In order to make this initiative operational and to prevent logistical delays, there must be well-developed mutual agreements between collaborating partner organizations in advance of an actual disaster to allow for quick deployment. A rigorous disaster education program provides AMC team members the knowledge base required for effective response and the skills to work more confidently in austere environments. Flexibility of the team's structure allows the AMC to respond quickly to evolving needs of requesting agencies, prevent institutional disruption, and sustain response. Complex human resource issues must be anticipated and addressed by the AMC's HR and risk management specialists. Finally, AMCs must anticipate and be willing and able to absorb some costs associated with the response, even when deploying with well-funded and highly resourced agencies.

REFERENCES

Babcock, Christine, Carolyn Baer, Jamil D. Bayram, Stacey Chamberlain, Jennifer L. Chan, Shannon Galvin, Jimin Kim, Melodie Kinet, Rashid F. Kysia, Janet Lin, Mamta Malik, Robert L. Murphy, Sola Olopade, and Christian Theodosis. 2010. "Chicago Medical Response to the 2010 Earthquake in Haiti: Translating Academic Collaboration into Direct Humanitarian Response." *Disaster Medicine and Public Health Preparedness* 4: 169-173.

Blackwell, Thomas, and Michael Bosse. 2007. "Use of an Innovative Design Mobile Hospital in the Medical Response to Hurricane Katrina." *Annals of Emergency Medicine* 49 (5): 580-588.

Brackbill, Robert M., Lorna E. Thorpe, Laura DiGrande, Megan Perrin, James H. Sapp, David Wu, Sharon Campolucci, Deborah J. Walker, Jim Cone, Paul Pulliam, Lisa Thalji, Mark R. Farfel, and Pauline Thomas. 2006. "Surveillance for World Trade Center Disaster Health Effects Among Survivors of Collapsed and Damaged Buildings." *MMWR Surveillance Summaries* 55 (2): 1-18.

Bryson, John M., Barbara C. Crosby, and Melissa M. Stone. 2006. "The Design and Implementation of Cross-sector Collaborations: Propositions from the Literature." *Public Administration Review* 66: 44-55.

FEMA. 2010. Emergency Management Institute. "IS-100HCb Introduction to the Incident Command System (ICS-100) for Healthcare/Hospitals." http://training.fema.gov/emiweb/is/is100b.asp (accessed July 9, 2011).

FEMA. 2011. Emergency Management Institute. "IS-700 National Incident Management System (NIMS), an Introduction." http://training.fema.gov/EMIWEB/IS/is700.asp (accessed July 9, 2011).

Gaudette, Ronald, Jay Schnitzer, Edward George, and Susan M. Briggs. 2002. "Lessons Learned from the September 11th World Trade Center Disaster: Pharmacy Preparedness and Participation in an International Medical and Surgical Response Team." *Pharmacotherapy* 22 (3): 271-281.

Ginzburg, Enrique, William O'Neill, Pascal J. Goldschmidt-Clermont, Eduardo de Marchena, Daniel Pust, and Barth A. Green. 2010. "Rapid Medical Relief—Project Medishare and the Haitian Earthquake." *New England Journal of Medicine* 362: e31. Epub February 24, 2010. PMID: 20181963.

Harrald, John R. 2006. "Agility and Discipline: Critical Success Factors for Disaster Response." *Annals of the American Academy of Political and Social Science* 604: 256-272.

Jobe, Kathleen. 2011. "Disaster Relief in Post-earthquake Haiti: Unintended Consequences of Humanitarian Volunteerism." *Travel Medicine and Infectious Diseases* 9 (1): 1-5. Epub December 3, 2010.

Kirsch, Thomas D., and Maggie R. Moon. 2010. "The line." *JAMA* 303 (10): 921-922.

Marklund, LeRoy A., Adrienne M. Graham, Patricia G. Morton, Charles G. Hurst, Ivette Motola, Donald W. Robinson, Vivian A. Kelley, Kimberly J. Elenberg, Michael F. Russler, Daniel E. Boehm, Dawn M. Higgins, Patrick E. McAndrew, Hope M. Williamson, Rodney D. Atwood, Kermit D. Heubner, Angel A. Brotons, Geoffrey T. Miller, Laukton Y. Rimpel, Larry L. Harris, Manuel Santiago, and LeRoy Cantrell. 2010. "Collaboration Between Civilian and Military Healthcare Professionals: A Better Way for Planning, Preparing, and Responding to All Hazard Domestic Events." Prehospital and Disaster Medicine 25 (5): 399-412.

McCunn, Maureen, Michael A. Ashburn, Thomas F. Floyd, C. William Schwab, Paul Harrington, C. William Hanson, Babak Sarani, Samir Mehta, Rebecca M. Speck, and Lee A. Fleisher. 2010. "An Organized, Comprehensive, and Security-enabled Strategic Response to the Haiti Earthquake: A Description of Pre-deployment Readiness Preparation and Preliminary Experience from an Academic Anesthesiology Department with No Preexisting International Disaster Response Program." *Anesthesia and Analgesia* 111 (6): 1438-1444. Epub September 14, 2010.

Medfilms Online, Inc. 2009.
http://www.medfilmsonline.com (accessed July 12, 2010).

National Disaster Life Support Foundation (NDLSF). 2007. "Course information page."
http://www.ndlsf.org/common/content.asp?PAGE=345 (accessed July 12, 2010).

Outward Bound Professional Programs. 2011.
http://www.outwardbound.org/index.cfm/do/cp.professional (accessed
July 12, 2010).

Schunk, Peggy K. 2009. "Hackensack University Medical Center
Demonstrates Its Disaster Response Readiness." Hackensack University
Medical Center press release, July 29.
http://www.humc.com/index.php?page=press&ev=1058 (accessed July 7, 2010).

Sklar, David P., Michael Richards, Mark Shah, and Paul Roth. 2007.
"Responding to Disasters: Academic Medical Centers' Responsibilities and
Opportunities." *Academic Medicine* 82: 797-800.

Subbarao, Italo, James M. Lyznicki, Edbert B. Hsu, Kristine M. Gebbie,
David Markenson, Barbara Barzansky, John H. Armstrong, Emmanuel
Cassimatis, Philip L. Coule, Cham E. Dallas, Richard V. King, Lewis
Rubinson, Richard Sattin, Raymond E. Swienton, Scott Lillibridge,
Frederick M. Burkle, Richard B. Schwartz, and James J. James. 2008. "A
Consensus-based Educational Framework and Competency Set for the
Discipline of Disaster Medicine and Public Health Preparedness." *Disaster
Medicine and Public Health Preparedness* 2: 57-68.

Thormar, Sigridur Bjork, Burthold Paul Rudolf Gersons, Barbara Juen,
Adelheid Marschang, Maria Nelden Djakababa, and Miranda Olff. 2010.
"The Mental Health Impact of Volunteering in a Disaster Setting: A
Review." *Journal of Nervous and Mental Disease* 198 (8): 529-538.

USAID. 2009. "Office of U.S. Foreign Disaster Assistance annual report for
fiscal year 2009."
http://www.usaid.gov/our_work/humanitarian_assistance/disaster_
assistance/publications/annual_reports/fy2009/annual_report_2009.pdf
(accessed February 3, 2011).

USAID. 2010. "Haiti—Earthquake Fact Sheet #48." Published April 2.
http://www.usaid.gov/our_work/humanitarian_assistance/disaster_
assistance/countries/haiti/template/fs_sr/fy2010/haiti_eq_fs48_04-02-
2010.pdf (accessed December 10, 2010).

Van Hoving, Daniel J., Lee A. Wallis, Fathima Docrat, and Shaheem De
Vries. 2010. "Haiti Disaster Tourism—A Medical Shame." *Prehospital and
Disaster Medicine* 25 (3): 201-202.

INTEROPERABILITY FOR FIRST RESPONDERS AND EMERGENCY MANAGEMENT: DEFINITION, NEED, AND THE PATH FORWARD

Kevin Thomas, *Boston University, School of Medicine*
Peter R. Bergethon, *Boston University, School of Medicine*
Mathew Reimer, *Boston University, School of Medicine*

INTRODUCTION

In the United States, the management of and response to a disaster usually involves multiple entities and organizations from the federal, state, and private sectors. Thus interoperability is important to successful disaster preparedness and response. The engineering definition of interoperability is "the ability of two or more systems or components to exchange information and to use the information that has been exchanged" (IEEE 1990). While this is a useful definition for infrastructures such as computers and telecommunications, it falls short in dealing with the human and organizational factors during a crisis response.

Crisis response encompasses technical, organizational, and cultural interoperability. Crises are unpredictable and endanger large segments of a population, often requiring focused or tailored responses. This creates the need for flexibility, preparedness, and adequately trained personnel capable of dealing with all-hazards events. Training should develop responders capable of rapidly assessing threats and acting accordingly, using ethical measures for mitigation, containment, and recovery.

Interoperability involves commonality of processes and technology, facilitating interactions between responders, stakeholders, and volunteers (Waugh and Streib 2006; Harrald 2006). Coordination through interoperability is necessary for efficient and timely crisis response. So far, developing the necessary process and infrastructure for crisis response has proven to be difficult (Waugh and Streib 2006).

The shared understanding across the many different first responder and emergency communities is more than a common language and information sharing protocols.

Unfortunately, the importance for interoperability is not fully understood by today's crisis managers. While most grasp the necessity for technological systems interoperability, there is insufficient appreciation of interoperable organizations and personnel. The scope of interoperability has been defined by Lerner et al. (2005) as "All aspects of collaboration and interaction needed to effectively prepare for, and respond to, disasters and other public health emergencies."

A robust relationship among the stakeholders should be encouraged and developed before a disaster occurs. It is unreasonable to expect that responders can merely be told to cooperate in order to achieve cooperation. Before a disaster occurs, operators from all relevant agencies must work together, building relationships and trust. Joint training during disaster drills and simulations, reaching across domains, are useful in developing a culture of interoperability.

Cultural changes must be made to operational guidelines to facilitate interoperability between individuals and agencies (Barbera and Olson 2004).

While executives may be willing to suggest that responders be more cooperative, they must also craft new policies and protocols that can enable that cooperation.

Integration will continue to be restrained across disciplines and regions as long as crisis responders are not privy to information pertaining to the total response capacity and situational awareness. This includes knowledge of transportation, patient care, medical supplies, and manpower assets that each provider may have at its disposal. Integration will remain elusive until active steps are taken to achieve transparent communication and information sharing between concerned participants. Integrated responses require collaboration between police, fire, emergency medical services, military responders, and public healthcare providers at all organizational levels. First responders from various agencies and jurisdictions must be able to reinforce each other to meet the challenges presented by different crises.

One of the greatest difficulties facing the crisis management community arises from the vertical and horizontal fragmentation in today's governing organizations (McConnell and Drennan 2006). Fragmentation fosters roadblocks to crisis planning and response. Horizontal fragmentation can be overcome through the development of interpersonal relationships between actors in the first responder community. The challenges presented by vertical fragmentation, however, require more formal solutions that address the organizational and cultural issues presented by different agencies. The response most likely to be successful is one that can utilize both an informal and a formal approach.

Another significant obstacle to interoperability is the reliance on government funding programs. Many funding programs are competitive and make it difficult to develop the relationships essential for interoperability. This adversarial culture is in direct contrast to collaboration and cooperation (Barbera and Olson 2004). The complexity of these obstacles brings to focus conflict between integrated contingency planning and the non-uniform realities of public, private, and government organizations (McConnell and Drennan 2006).

Political maneuvering, poorly defined command systems, and uncertainty about which roles and responsibilities are held by which organizations are also barriers to crisis response. They put emphasis on the need for a clear command structure, noting that ambiguity could cause significant disorder in a crisis, hindering effective response.

Training the first responder community effectively presents numerous difficulties (Livet et al. 2005). The great diversity across disciplines is one of the major causes of these difficulties. Impediments that arise from training individuals in highly specialized fields with differing levels of education and at times contradictory cultural ethics are formidable.

Along with the need to train first responders there is also the need to train the emergency management professionals from support organizations in fields such as finance and administration (Tierney 2007). All parties involved in a crisis must not only be trained to a high level of proficiency in their given field, but must also possess awareness of the other responders. Training should encompass all aspects of crisis planning, response, recovery, and mitigation (Tierney 2007).

Another benefit of training is increased awareness of the special needs of vulnerable populations. Examples are rehabilitation clinics and retirement facilities. The service providers to vulnerable populations will be better able to provide continued healthcare if they are aware of the timetable of response and just what external assistance can be expected (Stahmer et al. 2007).

By uniting all communities, there is a greater opportunity for mutual benefits to be derived. Interdisciplinary training may also assist healthcare providers in non-crisis situations such as immunizations, where responders can act as reserve healthcare providers in limited capacity. Also, through type-specific interdisciplinary training, such as violent situations, we can provide responders with the cross-agency awareness that has been identified as essential to effective crisis response (Vernon 2007).

Finally, it must be recognized that not every type of crisis can be anticipated. However, responders can be made ready to address these through effective training. The key to successful crisis management and response is the creation of cross-discipline and interagency integrated response. Responsible organizations at the federal and state levels should provide resources and opportunities and promulgate policies to ensure interoperability training and teamwork in disaster response.

REFERENCES

Barbera, Joseph, and Laura Olson. 2004. "Report on the First Regional EMS Forum." *National Capitol Area,* July 6.

Harrald, John R. 2006. "Agility and Discipline: Critical Success Factors for Disaster Response." *Annals of the American Academy of Political and Social Science* 604 (*Shelter from the Storm: Repairing the National Emergency Management System after Hurricane Katrina*) (March): vol. 604(1):256-272.

Institute of Electrical and Electronics Engineers (IEEE). 1990. *IEEE Standard Computer Dictionary: A Compilation of IEEE Standard Computer Glossaries.* New York: IEEE.

Lerner, E. Brooke, Anthony J. Billittier IV, Robert E. O'Connor, Michael P. Allswede, Thomas H. Blackwell, Henry E. Wang, and Lynn J. White. 2005. "Linkages of Acute Care and EMS to State and Local Public Health Programs: Application to Public Health Programs." *Journal of Public Health Management Practice* 11 (4): 291-297.

Livet, Melanie, Jane Richter, LuAnne Ellison, Bill Dease, Lawrence McClure, Charles Feigley, and Donna L. Richter. 2005. "Emergency Preparedness Academy Adds Public Health to Readiness Equation." *Journal of Public Health Management & Practice* (November/December Supplement). 11(6): S4-S10.

McConnell, Allan, and Lynn Drennan. 2006. "Mission Impossible? Planning and Preparing for Crisis." *Journal of Contingencies and Crisis Management* 14 (2): 59-70.

Stahmer, S.A., S.R. Ellison, K.K. Jubanyik, S. Felten, C. Doty, L. Binder, and N.J. Jouriles. 2007. "Integrating the Core Competencies: Proceedings from the 2005 Academic Assembly Consortium." *Academic Emergency Medicine* 14 (1) (January): 80-94.

Tierney, Kathleen J. 2007. "Testimony on Needed Emergency Management Reforms." Journal of Homeland Security and Emergency Management 4 (3): Article 15.

Vernon, August. 2007. "Fire-EMS Response to Mass Shootings: If There Were a Report of a Mass Shooting in Your Community, How Would You Respond?" *Firehouse Magazine* 32 (6) (June): 58(3). http://find.galegroup.com.ezproxy.bu.edu/itx/start.do?prodId=ITOF (accessed November 1, 2007).

Waugh, William L. Jr., and Gregory Streib. 2006. "Collaboration and Leadership for Effective Emergency Management." *Public Administration Review* 66 (s1): 131-140.

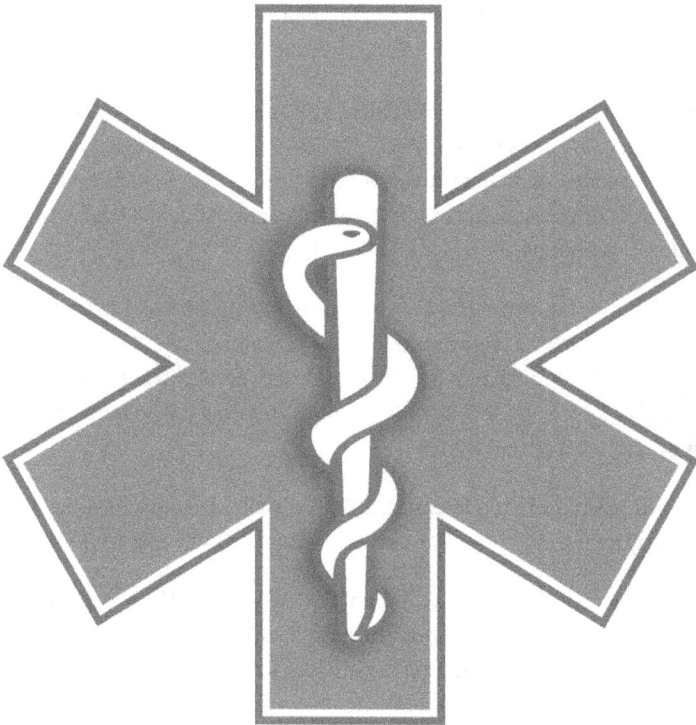

THE USE OF U.S. ACADEMIC INSTITUTIONS IN COMMUNITY MEDICAL DISASTER RECOVERY

Arnauld Nicogossian, *George Mason University*
Thomas Zimmerman, *Palm Beach Medical College, Florida*
Gloria Addo-Ayensu, *Fairfax County Health Department*
Kevin Thomas, *Boston University, School of Medicine*
Gary L. Kreps, *George Mason University*
Nelya Ebadirad, *George Mason University*
Sulava Gautam, *George Mason University*

INTRODUCTION

Communities prone to disasters are more likely to develop and exercise preparedness plans (Graham et al. 2006). Proactive disaster preparedness is essential to improve emergency management for all community assets, including schools (Shelton, Owens, and Song 2009). Schools are designed to accommodate hundreds of students and provide a learning experience in a healthy and safe environment (Department of Homeland Security 2010). They have certain physical attributes of interest to disaster planners and policymakers. Schools operate cafeterias, have janitorial services, manage a transportation system (school vans and buses), and possess large, open spaces such as playgrounds and exercise facilities. School locations, like other civic areas, are familiar to parents and other community residents. They can and on occasion have been used as nodes for mass vaccination, drug distribution, prescreening patients, psychological counseling, temporary shelters, and quarantine. Post-disaster triage and outpatient care can be set up on school premises (Gebhart and Pence 2007).

Utilizing schools for disaster preparedness is not a new concept. In 2008 Hurricane Ike devastated coastal regions of the Gulf of Mexico. The Birdville Independent School District (BISD), Texas and the United States promptly responded by opening shelters in two high and two middle schools (BISD 2008). Victims of Hurricane Katrina were evacuated and relocated across the United States. The Wanamaker Junior High Schools in Philadelphia housed 54 Hurricane Katrina survivors and cared for 130 evacuees, providing resources such as communication, food, and healthcare services (Drexel University School of Public Health 2010). The American Red Cross (ARC) has executed agreements with the U.S. Federal Emergency Management Agency (FEMA) and individual state education authorities for the use of schools in disaster recovery and medical support (Department of Education N.Y. State 2010; American Red Cross 2010).

A U.S. federal legislation promoting school security and safety, including the development of emergency communications networks, has been enacted following the Columbine, Colorado school massacre (Crime Awareness and Campus Security Act). This legislation was initially backed by grants, which were curtailed in the 2010–2011 appropriation budgets. The Department of Homeland Security published a report stating that in the aftermath of disasters, intact schools were used to help community recovery efforts (Department of Homeland Security 2010).

There are 98,916 public schools in the United States comprising elementary schools, middle schools, and high schools, which enroll 55 million students from kindergarten to 12th grade (The Center for Education Reform 2009; Graham et al. 2006). The responsibility for protecting and ensuring the safety of such a large segment of the U.S. population is complex and the current study investigators assumed that this experience can benefit community medical disaster preparedness and recovery.

METHODOLOGY

The preliminary assessment of the utility of public schools, and other academic institutions, to community medical disaster preparedness and recovery was limited to four specific inquiries:

1. Use of school infrastructure (physical facilities) and services.

2. School ability to function as educational and communication nodes using existing educational and outreach capacity.

3. Ethical and legal concerns of assigning schools a non-traditional and dual role.

4. Potential contributions of other local community infrastructure to enhance schools utility.

The study approach consisted of literature reviews, spatial and geographic relationship of the schools in the Northern Virginia (NOVA) region with communities, and a subject-matter expert's workshop addressing the four issues under investigation. All information was combined to produce a final assessment. The following five steps summarize this approach:

(1) Literature acquisition, selection, and pre-screening of abstracts.

(2) Literature evaluation for the strength of evidence.

(3) Geographic Information System (GIS) analysis to address the spatial relationships of schools to communities and other infrastructures in the NOVA region. The GIS methodology used to identify the NOVA region schools relationship to resources has been described in previous publications (Zook et al. 2010; Koizumi 2010).

(4) Discussions of issues by subject-matter experts.

(5) Integration of steps (1)–(4).

The literature acquisition and review methodology has been detailed in a recent publication (Nicogossian et al. 2010). Literature searches were conducted using Medical Subject Heading (MeSH) terms (National Center for Biotechnology Information 2010) to query search engines such as Medline, Cochrane Collaboration, and Google Scholar. Primary MeSH terms included schools and university infrastructure and facilities, disasters planning and recovery for schools, school-based disaster response for medical community needs, legislations and academic facilities for disaster-response and medical preparedness, ethical aspects for the use in a dual role of the educational facilities, academic facilities as shelters and medical triage units, communications, etc.

Each abstract and website was pre-screened for relevance to the topic under investigation. Selected publications and materials were evaluated using the subjective and qualitative approach described in Table 1.

Table 1. Subjective and Qualitative Categorization of Literature Strength

Strenght Level	Explanation	Justification
1	Good Evidence	Scientifically validated information with minimal experimental bias, or benefits that outweigh the risks
2	Fair Evidence	Limited scientific information with potential for bias, or potential benefits that outweigh the risks
3	Inconclusive Evidence	Expert opinion and/or limited scientific information with potential for significant bias and/or benefits do not outweigh the risks
4	Evidence Lacking	No scientific information and/or risks outweigh benefits

RESULTS

Literature Acquisition and Evaluation

The literature search yielded no meta-analysis or randomized control trials. Sixty publications were identified and screened for relevance. From those, 12 (including two books) were selected for further in-depth evaluations. A strength level 2 was assigned to all nine refereed publications.[1] Books and websites providing specific information, or case studies, on the use of schools in disasters were categorized as level 3, with the remaining government reports and websites rated as level 4. None of the materials accessed met the level 1 criterion.

There is fair evidence that structurally safe schools can be used for medical disaster recovery. A 2004 survey of more than 2,100 school system superintendents found that only 86% did develop a disaster-response plan. Almost 95% of school administrators had an evacuation plan, but 30% had never conducted an evacuation drill. The same study finds that 22% did not have disaster plans accommodating children with special needs, and 25% lacked plans for post-disaster counseling (Johnston and Redlener 2006). School preparedness to handle students and staff can serve as an indicator of the readiness and ability (Aburto et al. 2010; Beaton et al. 2007; Elder and Crespo 2010; Gebhart and Pence 2007; Graham et al. 2006; Johnston and Redlener 2006; Maher, Price, and Zirkel 2010; Shelton, Owens, and Song 2009; Stuber et al. 2002) to support community needs and should be investigated further.

Fair evidence supports the fact that most urban school districts are better equipped for disaster response than rural districts (Graham et al. 2006). Fair evidence also supports the fact that in the aftermath of disasters, the majority of public schools are usually closed and unused. From August to December 2009, there were at least 1,947 school closures due to the 2009 A(H1N1) pandemic influenza threats. During the two waves—a period of approximately 96 school days—3,298 schools were closed for one or more days. From April to June 2010, 1,351 schools (1% of schools nationwide) from 34 states and the District of Columbia dismissed all students for at least one day (The Office of Safe Drug-Free Schools, U.S. Department of Education 2007). With proper planning, closed schools can serve community recovery needs without further disruption of classes.

During Hurricane Andrew, Florida schools were made inoperable (Provenzo, Eugene, and Fradd 1995). The Northridge earthquake damaged local schools and universities in California. After the Red River flooded in the spring of 1997, North Dakota and Minnesota schools were swamped by mud and made unusable (Federal Emergency Management Agency 2010). Hurricanes Katrina and Rita heavily impacted Louisiana's schools. Nearly 176,000 students were displaced, including more than 72,000 who left the state. In New Orleans alone, the storms closed 71 schools (Louisiana Recovery Authority 2010).

In response to Hurricane Katrina, Tulane University closed and evacuated over 400 students to the Jackson State University in Mississippi. The Tulane University Hospital and its clinics continued to serve patients from the region despite the loss of power (Carey 2006) and until evacuation was feasible.

The use of schools to provide psychological assistance and crisis counseling is common after traumatic events (The Office of Safe Drug-Free Schools, U.S. Department of Education 2007). In the aftermath of September 11, 2001, more than half of the students undergoing counseling after the attack received it through schools (Stuber et al. 2002). Furthermore, schools are available to non-governmental organizations (NGOs) such as the American Red Cross for counseling and as distribution centers (American Red Cross 2010).

GIS Analysis of the NOVA Region

The NOVA region served as a case study to model the distribution and spatial relationship of schools and community resources for medical disaster preparedness and recovery. The association among schools, strip malls, and healthcare facilities identified disparities among NOVA counties/cities. In general, eastern counties and cities in more densely populated areas have better access to such facilities than the western region. GIS analysis also showed that strip malls and schools are more likely to coexist in the densely populated eastern region. GIS analysis of the NOVA revealed that there are fewer hospitals than schools:

635 schools and only 16 hospitals and healthcare centers. Most medical facilities are, however, located within three miles of a school, which could serve as a satellite triage or first-aid center operated by the hospital staff and prevent against sudden outpatient surge capacity.

An assessment of the walking accessibility of schools in the NOVA region indicated that schools are located close to main roads; however, some schools are not within walking distance for all community members. Additionally, up to 90% of the population is located within a one-mile (1.609 km) radius and 97% within a three-mile radius from a school buffer zone (4.828 km).

Discussions by Subject-Matter Experts

Fairfax County and the rest of NOVA are susceptible to a variety of natural hazards, including floods, hurricanes, and tornadoes, and human-made disasters such as hazardous waste spills and terrorist attacks (Fairfax County 2010). Subject-matter experts represented a wide range of organizations from the United States and Canada.[2] The discussions focused primarily on the NOVA experience, specifically the Fairfax County region. No consensus was sought during the workshop. Individual conclusions are summarized below:

(a) Fairfax County Public Schools (FCPS) has a close collaboration with local, state, and federal health, safety, and emergency management organizations to develop plans for emergency crisis mitigation (Fairfax County Public Schools 2010a).

(b) The experience gained from the collaborative efforts between the FCPS and the NOVA Fairfax County Health Department (FCHD) can benefit community resiliency (Fairfax County Public Schools 2010a).

(c) Schools allow access for ground and air logistics and can be used as shelters or first-aid stations. Most urban schools are also located in the vicinity of services such as restaurants, pharmacies, urgent care centers, veterinary clinics, and medical professional buildings. These services usually are part of strip malls and conceptually can serve as additional temporary disaster-response resources.

(d) Use of GIS analysis can help identify and allocate resources.

(e) Sources for liability insurance and ethical considerations should be an important consideration in planning for school use during community medical disaster preparedness and recovery.

DISCUSSION

Many U.S. and international guidelines mention the possible utility of schools for medical disaster preparedness and recovery (Action Aid International 2010). The importance of education in promoting and enabling the use of schools in disasters has been emphasized (Institute of Development Studies 2010). Most U.S. states require schools to prepare for disasters. There is a fundamental link between day-to-day emergency readiness and disaster recovery. Some schools have introduced disaster reduction education into their curricula to raise awareness and provide a better understanding of disaster management by students, teachers, and communities (Regional Consultative Committee 2007). Improving building codes and structural hardening can increase the safety of buildings, protect students and staff, and serve the community following disasters. Investing in hardening school infrastructures and/or stockpiling survival and emergency gear should be assessed for cost/benefit tradeoffs (USA Today 2010; International Strategy for Disaster Reduction 2006). Recent federal budget cuts will probably affect schools security programs and perhaps their utility to community disaster preparedness (Beaton et al. 2007).

Since 2004 FEMA has provided grants to universities for developing training programs for disaster preparedness and improving community resiliency (CTGP 2010). Many colleges and universities that are recipients of disaster preparedness grants, including George Mason University (GMU), did establish an emergency preparedness office and regularly exercise an all-hazards response plan (Federal Emergency Management Agency 2008). These assets could be amplified and linked to community preparedness as a whole.

Local, state, and federal authorities must consider the potential risks and shortcomings of transforming school staff into community first responders without proper training and support. The results of literature reviews were inconclusive on the use of school staff, specifically the services, maintenance, and healthcare personnel, for community disaster relief.

The benefits and risks of using schools as alternative public health/ medical resources in disaster preparedness and recovery should be carefully vetted by local, state, and federal authorities. For example, during the 2009 influenza, lack of vaccines precluded the use of schools for mass vaccination (Aburto et al. 2010).

Liability insurance is important in disaster planning. While all schools hold liability insurance, this insurance only covers medical costs for a student's injury resulting from school negligence. Organizations and community members are allowed to use school infrastructure for civic purposes, such as after-hours meetings and training. These groups have to present proof of insurance since most schools cannot afford liability insurance to cover such civic functions (Fairfax County Public Schools 2010b). Ethical considerations should be included into the process of medical policies formulation. Community concerns should be addressed during the planning process to improve compliance with policies and prevent confusion in the roles and responsibilities of schools (Maher, Price, and Zirkel 2010).

Evidence-based research targeting practice guidelines should be carried out to further refine the proper role and needs of schools in community medical disaster preparedness and recovery.

POLICY IMPLICATIONS AND CONCLUSIONS

Schools should be considered as part of all community activities involving medical disaster planning and resiliency. With adequate financing and logistic support from local, state, and federal governments, schools could be a viable and successful community asset following disasters.

This preliminary review identified a potential benefit from including local universities, especially those that do have undergraduate and graduate medical training as an important educational resource to support schools in medical disaster preparedness, response, and recovery. Universities, although also resource constrained, possess assets that can be readily adapted to support communities and perhaps serve as hubs for local schools' educational and outreach networks.

Many natural disasters, such as earthquakes, storms, and floods, can impact and even destroy community infrastructures. As a result, these disasters could impede the use of schools in the affected area. Schools have been used as alternative medical facilities in a limited number of disaster scenarios. These scenarios primarily include epidemics and human-made biological disasters. Hardening school infrastructure and implementing new legislation aimed at improving the building codes to withstand different types of disasters should be a major policy consideration. Hardening school infrastructure might not be enough to protect them from devastating disasters such as floods, earthquakes, and hurricanes.

Table 2 is an attempt to summarize the complex and multi-dimensional relationships between schools and the different types of disasters. A 1–5 Likert Scale (1 representing the highest score) was used to relate the functional capacity of schools to individual disasters. These rankings must be validated with additional research and studies.

Table 2. Use of Schools in Disaster Preparedness and Recovery

Type §	Sub-type	Disaster	Extent *	Duration **	School Integrity***	Accessibility by Roads	Availability for Use	Building Code	Rank *****
NATURAL	Geothermal	Earthquake Tsunami Volcanic eruption	Multiregional	Several hours to <1 week	No*	May not be accessible†	UA****	Yes (new location)	5
	Topological	Landslides Avalanches Wild fires	Multiregional	Hours but <1 day	No	May not be accessible†	UA	No (better site selection)	5
	Hydrometeoro-logical	Hurricanes Tornadoes Flood/ drought	Multiregional	Minutes to days	Maybe	May not be accessible†	AA‡	Yes	5
	Biological	Epidemics Pandemics	Multiregional	Days to months depending on the agent	Yes	Accessible†	AA	N/A	1
HUMAN-MADE	Technological	Explosion Leakage Pollution	Local/Multiregional	Minutes to days (contamination)	No	May not be accessible†	UA	N/A (air filtering system)	3
	Transportation	Air/land/sea disaster	Local	Minutes to hours	Yes	Accessible†	AA	Proximity to hazard	N/A
	Structure Collapse	Mine/bridge collapse	Local	Minutes to days	Maybe	May not be accessible†	AA	N/A	3
	Production Failure	Computer system breakdown	Multiregional	Minutes to days (contamination)	N/A	N/A	N/A	N/A	N/A
	Conflict	War (traditional or non-traditional) Siege	Local/Multiregional	Days to years	No	Unsafe	AA	N/A	5

*Denotes spread and affected area up to 100 miles or more

**Denotes length of time the hazard is devastating the area

***Denotes the ability of the structure to maintain integrity and functionality

****Unaffected area (UA): emphasizes that only schools located outside of disaster areas might be usable as distribution centers, makeshift hospitals, etc.

*****Defines school usability in the affected area, with 1 being highly recommended and 5 not recommended

†May not be accessible due to extent of destruction. Air access might be possible

‡AA stands for affected area

§Adapted from the National Oceanographic and Atmospheric Agency 2010

NOTES

1. Aburto et al. (2010), Beaton et al. (2007), Elder and Crespo (2010), Gebhart and Pence (2007), Graham et al. (2006), Johnston and Redlener (2006), Maher, Price, and Zirkel (2010), Shelton, Owens, and Song (2009), and Stuber et al. (2002).

2. American Red Cross, Fairfax County Public Schools (FCPS), the Fairfax County Health Department (FCHD), George Mason University, Boston University, Inova Health System, McMaster University, New York Presbyterian Hospital Center, National Center for Disaster Medicine and Public Health (NCDMPH), Uniform Services University, Centers for Disease Control and Prevention (CDC), Hospital Corporation of America, and Public Schools Risk Institute, Inc.

This pilot study was supported by a competitive grant from George Mason University. The authors wish to thank the following experts for their thoughtful inputs and critiques: Heidi Cordi MD, MPH, Columbia Presbyterian Hospital; Lisa Eckenwiler PhD, Healthcare Ethics and Center for Health Policy Research and Ethics—GMU; Fred Ellis BS, Fairfax County Public Schools—Office of Safety and Security; Daniel Hanfling MD, Emergency Management and Disaster Medicine, INOVA Health System; David McCann MD, McMaster University; Kenneth Schor DO, MPH, National Center for Disaster Medicine and Public Health; Franceska Schroeder Esq., Fish & Richardson P.C., and Edward Septimus MD, Hospital Corporation of America.

REFERENCES

Aburto, N.J., et al. 2010. "Knowledge and Adoption of Community Mitigation Efforts in Mexico During the 2009 H1N1 Pandemic." *American Journal of Preventative Medicine* 39 (5): 395-402.

Action Aid International. 2010. "Disaster Risk Reduction Through Schools." http://www.actionaid.org/assets/pdf/disaster-through-schools.pdf.

American Red Cross. 2010. "Disaster Services." http://www.redcrosslv.org/disaster.html.

American Red Cross press release. 2010. www.nvoad.org/index.php/rl/doc.../16moa-red-cross-and-arc.html.

Beaton, R., et al. 2007. *Biosecurity and Bioterrorism: Biodefense Strategy, Practice, and Science* 5 (4): 327-334.

BISD. 2008. "BISD Schools Provide Shelter for Hurricane Ike Evacuees." *Inside BISD*, September 24. http://www.bryanisd.org/docs/InsideBISD 092408.pdf.

Carey, B. 2006. *Leave No One Behind: Hurricane Katrina and the Rescue of Tulane Hospital.* Nashville: Clearbrook Press.

Department of Education N.Y. State. 2010. "Schools, Shelters, and The Red Cross." www.p12.nysed.gov/facplan/Emergency/sheltermanagerarticle.html

Department of Homeland Security. 2010. "School Safety." http://www.dhs.gov/ files/programs/gc_1183486267373.shtm.

Drexel University School of Public Health. 2010. "Katrina Relief Efforts." http://publichealth.drexel.edu/News/News_Archive_2005/Katrina_Relief_Efforts/158/.

Elder, J.P., and N.C. Crespo. 2010. "Community Mitigation of Disease Outbreaks: Health Communication Perspectives." *American Journal of Preventative Medicine* 39 (5): 487-488.

Fairfax County. 2010. "Fairfax County Pre-Disaster Recovery Plan." http://www.fairfaxcounty.gov/oem/pdrp/.

Fairfax County Public Schools. 2010a. "Emergency Preparedness and Support." http://www.fcps.edu/emergencyplan/.

Fairfax County Public Schools. 2010b. "Risk Management."
http://www.fcps.edu/fs/budget/riskmanagement/.

Federal Emergency Management Agency. 2008. "DHS Awards $63 Million in
Emergency Preparedness Grants."
http://www.fema.gov/news/newsrelease.fema?id=45733.

Federal Emergency Management Agency. 2010. "How Schools Can Become
More Disaster Resistant." http://www.fema.gov/kids/schdizr.htm.

Gebhart, M.E., and R. Pence. 2007. "START Triage: Does it Work?" *Disaster
Management and Response* 5 (3): 68-73.

Graham et al. 2006. "Mass-casualty Events at Schools: A National
Preparedness Survey." *Pediatrics* 117 (1): 8-15.

Institute of Development Studies. 2010. "Role of Education and Schools in
Disaster Risk Reduction."
http://www.eldis.org/go/topics/resourceguides/climate-change/key-issues/
children/-climate-change-anddisasters/role-of-education-and-schools-in-
disaster-risk-reduction.

International Strategy for Disaster Reduction. 2006. "Keynote Address by
Sálvano Briceño."
http://www.unisdr.org/preventionweb/files/5609_speechHarvard.pdf.

Johnston, C., and I. Redlener. 2006. "Critical Concepts for Children in Disasters
Identified by Hands-on Professionals: Summary of Issues Demanding
Solutions Before the Next One." *Pediatrics* 117 (5 pt 3): S458-S460.

Koizumi, N. 2010. "Geographic Disparity in Access to Organ Transplant
in the United States and Other Western Countries." *World Medical and
Health Policy* 2 (6): 111-131.

Louisiana Recovery Authority. 2010. "Task Forces."
http://www.lra.louisiana.gov/ index.cfm?md=pagebuilder&tmp=home&ni
d=34&pnid=0&pid=91&fmid =0&catid=0&elid=0&ssid=0.

Maher, P.J., K. Price, and P.A. Zirkel. 2010. "Governmental and Official
Immunity for School Districts and their Employees: Alive and Well?"
Kansas Journal of Law and Public Policy 19 (2): 234-268.

National Center for Biotechnology Information. 2010. "MeSH."
www.ncbi.nlm. nih.gov/mesh.

Nicogossian, A.N., et al. 2010. "Influenza Immunization: Synthesizing and Communicating the Evidence." *World Medical & Health Policy* 2 (2): 5184.

Provenzo J.R., F. Eugene, and S.H. Fradd. 1995. *Hurricane Andrew, The Public Schools, and the Rebuilding of Community*. Albany: State of New York Press.

Regional Consultative Committee. 2007. "Integrating Disaster Risk Reduction into School Curriculum: Mainstreaming Disaster Risk Reduction into Education." http://www.ineesite.org/assets/ADPCIntegratingDRRIntoSchoolCurriculu m.pdf.

Shelton, A.J., E.W. Owens, and H. Song. 2009. "An Examination of Public School Safety Measures across Geographic Settings." *Journal of School Health* 79 (1): 24-29.

Stuber, J., et al. 2002. "Determinants of Counseling for Children in Manhattan after the September 11 Attacks." *Psychiatric Services* 53 (7): 815-822.

The Center for Education Reform. 2009. "K-12 Facts." http://www.edreform.com/ Fast_Facts/K12_Facts/.

The Office of Safe Drug-Free Schools, U.S. Department of Education. 2007. "Practical Information on Crisis Planning: A Guide for Schools and Communities." http://www2.ed.gov/admins/lead/safety/emergencyplan/crisisplanning.pdf.

USA Today. 2010. "Flood Insurance Claims." http://www.usatoday.com/news/nation/2010-08-25-flood-insurance_N.htm.

Zook, M., et al. 2010. "Volunteered Geographic Information and Crowdsourcing Disaster Relief: A Case Study of the Haitian Earthquake." *World Medical and Health Policy* 2 (2): 7-33.

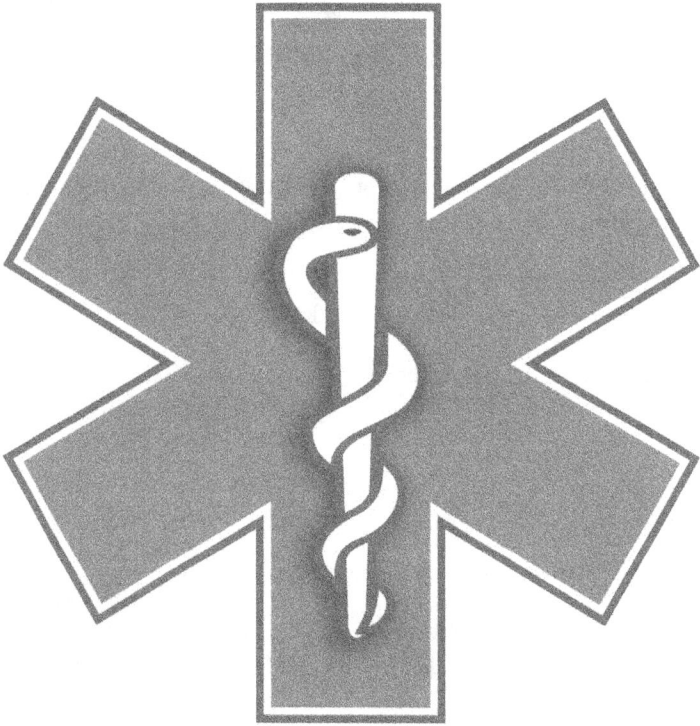

A PHYSICIAN'S REMEMBRANCE OF 9-11: WHERE WE WERE AND WHERE WE ARE

Heidi P. Cordi, *The New York Presbyterian Hospital*

INTRODUCTION

On September 7, 2001, I remember being on the 23rd floor of Tower 7 of the World Trade Center, visiting New York City's (NYC's) Office of Emergency Management (OEM). OEM was created by Mayor Giuliani in 1996 to manage NYC's response to events such as terrorism. I was visiting as an invited guest in preparation for Operation TriPOD (Trial Point of Dispensing), a drill for distribu-tion of medication in the event of a biological attack. I was particularly amazed at how thick the OEM walls were, and to look out of the window was like looking down a long narrow corridor, until you could catch a glimpse of the City That Never Sleeps, with its massive communications systems that would be deployed "if something happened." I stood there and wondered…"what if?" because in my mind, I was already preparing for an emergency egress. How fast could I run down 23 flights? Little did I realize that just four days later, the unimaginable would happen.

The NYC Office of Emergency Management (OEM) has certainly come a long way since 1950, during the Cold War when it was known as the Office for Civilian Defense (OCD) and was preparing for an atomic attack. Ironically, it was to also help residents prepare for an enemy air attack and coordinate civil defense programs with nearby counties and cities. Under Title III of the Federal Super-fund Amendments and Reauthorization Act of 1986, each locality is required to organize a Local Emergency Planning Committee (LEPC).

NYC OEM had regular drills and disaster scenarios with respective agen-cies and stakeholders. Many scenarios were based on previous disasters such as the sarin gas attack, anthrax attacks, truck bombs, bubonic plague, and even a simulated plane crash. Operation TriPOD was administered by NYC OEM in co-operation with U.S. Department of Justice, Weill Cornell Medical College of Cornell Medical Center, NYC Department of Health (DOH), NYC Fire Depart-ment, NY Police Department, American Red Cross, and 600 volunteers. It was scheduled for September 12, 2001.

On September 11, 2001, we learned that our U.S. borders were not safe, our Nation's security was at risk, and that we were vulnerable. I also learned that my fears had come true. Why did it take September 11, 2001, to be a wake-up call? Although the U.S. Government has held numerous top-secret exercises (aka disaster preparedness?) for potential terrorist threats for two decades, this horrific event was not averted. Throughout the 1980s, there were several Continuity of Government (COG) exercises that rehearsed how to keep the federal government running during and after a nuclear war with the Soviet Union. Even after the fall of the Soviet Union, the United States continued with its exercises about possible terrorist attacks, but this time against U.S. soil (Mann 2004). Sometime between 1991 and 2001, a regional sector of the North American Aerospace Defense Command simulated a foreign hijacked airliner crashing into a building in the United States as part of a training exercise scenario (Clarke 2004). After Presiden-tial Decision Directive 39 (PDD-39) was issued in June 1995 requiring key feder-al agencies to maintain well-exercised counterterrorist capabilities, many more training exercises were conducted between 1995 and 1998 across the United States based on potential terrorist events involving aircraft hijackings and weap-ons of mass destruction (U.S. General Accounting Office 1999).

Ironically, on September 11, 2001, the military was conducting one of its yearly exercises called Global Guardian (which is a global readiness exer-cise in-volving all Stratcom forces and aims to test the military's command and control procedures in the event of a nuclear attack) in conjunction with

Vigilant Guardian (the annual training exercise conducted by NORAD in which a threat to North American airspace is simulated) (Arkin 2005). This exercise was a postulated bomber attack from the former Soviet Union on North America according to The 9/11 Commission Report (National Commission on Terrorist Attacks upon the United States 2004).

WHAT HAPPENED IN THE LAST DECADE SINCE THAT FATEFUL DAY?

TriPOD did eventually take place on May 22, 2002, and served as a poignant re-minder that preparedness for any disaster is imperative, because we were once again terrorized just a few months after 9/11, this time with the biologic weapon, anthrax.

The federal government selected NYC as the site of several "research" and development projects pertinent to disaster preparedness. The following are just a few highlights from NYC OEM Biennial Reports (New York City Office of Emergency Management 2005; 2007).

Urban Dispersion Program. In March 2004, the first of three scientific field stud-ies in a program known as the Urban Dispersion Program (UDP) were conducted near Madison Square Garden. UDP aims to monitor the release and dispersion of harmless gases in the canyons of New York (the space between our large sky-scrapers) in order to gather data to improve the accuracy of plume modeling in major metropolitan areas throughout the country.

National Atmospheric Release Advisory Center (NARAC). NARAC provides New York access to sophisticated, satellite-based plume model-ing capabilities that pro-vide immediate, real-time airflow prediction and consequence management in re-sponse to the release of any traceable airborne hazardous materials.

Regional Radiological Pilot Program. OEM led the design and devel-opment of a regional radiological detection and monitoring system that included the installa-tion of a regional detection data integration system and provided a model for other regional efforts throughout the country.

BioWatch, a Department of Homeland Security program, provides the City with air collectors that sample for biological agents.

Operation United Response was a major field exercise at Shea Stadium (Citi-Field) designed to test the City's ability to respond to a "weapons of mass destruc-tion" attack on a stadium or another large public venue.

Operation Transit SAFE was inspired by the Madrid Bombings and was the City's first interagency subway exercise, held in May 2004. Funded by the De-partment of Homeland Security, the Operation was conducted at lower Manhat-tan's Bowling Green subway station and tested the City's response to a terrorist attack in the subway system.

PODEX, held in 2005, was a two-part exercise designed to test the City's mass prophylaxis and logistical response to a biological event. This exercise included a live test of the capability of the City's mass prophylaxis point of dispensing pro-gram (POD) and our ability to activate and deliver medica-tions contained in the Strategic National Stockpile to specific dispensing sites in New York City. Center for Disease Control had set forth the goal that every person should receive prophylaxis within a 48-hour time-frame.

Additionally, NYC OEM has been helping to prepare its citizens for disas-ters in a "Ready New York" preparedness campaign since 2003 with print and electronic publications in nine languages, public service announcements, print and outdoor advertising, a speaker's bureau, corporate partnerships, and hands-on preparedness training programs.

In 2005, the protocol document for the Citywide Incident Management System (CIMS) was implemented. This was to be New York City's program for responding to and recovering from emergencies, and for managing planned events working closely with NYC emergency service agencies while work-ing closely with City, State, private, and not-for-profit agencies and entities.

New York City has conducted 22 exercises in the last 10 years.

We also learned that businesses, including hospitals, must be able to run unimpeded (Kayyem and Chang 2002). Although risk and threat assessments help to guide disaster preparedness (e.g., low probability of a hurricane hitting Sioux Falls), hospitals need to be equally prepared for any potential terror event as even they are not immune. Terrorists even targeted two hospitals in 2008 in Ahmeda-bad, India, where injured people were brought after they suffered injuries at a previous bombing (The Times of India 2008).

Are we, 10 years after September 11, any better prepared for "the next ter-rorist attack?" Just as terrorists know no boundaries, they may also know that just when we are not looking, or not thinking about it, they will strike. It is easy to schedule a drill in advance, but when the actual event occurs, are we ready? There is no national requirement for hospitals to have particular disaster plans (Lord and Bogis 2010). Although there was a program that started after 9/11 to help hospi-tals purchase some of the necessary items needed during a disaster, it, like many preparedness programs, has been cut from the federal budget. We encourage self-preparedness (72-hour self-sustaining); however, we cannot expect those who are injured, disabled, or dependent to be able to take care of themselves. The injured will inevitably seek medical attention, as well as those "worried well." We must be able to take care of everyone and build medical resiliency. Yet, if there were a chemical, biological, radiological, or nuclear (CBRN) attack, could the already overcrowded hospitals and their Emergency Departments handle the anticipated massive surge of patients even though they have developed a working draft on Surge Capacity? The demand on the medical system is already taxing. It is hard to even imagine.

The New York City Department of Health and Mental Hygiene has a Healthcare Emergency Preparedness Program (HEPP). They collaborate on mul-tiple initiatives with a variety of healthcare providers and facilities, including hos-pitals, primary care clinics, long-term care facilities, emergency medical services, medical schools, professional associations, and agencies, and further enhance NYC's emergency readiness. The primary source of funding for these activities is the federal agency, the Health Resources Services Administration. Each hospital is required to conduct two Emergency Management/Emergency Operations Plans, one of which can be a table-top exercise; the other must also include an "influx of simulated patients," according to the Joint Commission on Accreditation of Healthcare Organizations.

There have been a multitude of programs and protocol changes that have affected the way we now prepare in New York City, especially since September 11, 2001. Each disaster we face, whether "planned" or reality, makes me feel maybe a little more secure in our efforts to be able to take care of ourselves "in case of an emergency." After all, the mission of Homeland Security is to take care of the Homeland, we need to be able to take care of ourselves.

Terrorism is now a part of our lives, even in our own backyard. We have now integrated responses to its potential occurrence into everyday living, whether it is by getting to the airport at least two hours earlier than our designated flight, or how we practice emergency preparedness at hospitals. No longer will we be vulnerable, nor will we hide. It was an emotional and financial toll that turned our daily lives around forever on September 11, 2001. Will these plans ever really work? I hope we never have to find out.

REFERENCES

Arkin, William M. 2005. "Code Names Deciphering US Military Plans, Programs, and Operations in the 9/11 World." http://books.google.com/books?id=KXLfAAAAMAAJ.

Clarke, Richard A. 2004. *Against All Enemies: Inside America's War on Terror.* New York: Free Press.

Kayyem, Juliette N., and Patricia E. Chang. 2002. "Beyond Business Continuity: The Role of the Private Sector in Preparedness Planning." Belfer Center for Science and International Affairs Harvard University. http://belfercenter.ksg.harvard.edu/files/beyond%20business%20continuity.pdf (accessed July 25, 2011).

Lord, Gregg, and Arnold Bogis. 2010. "Supply and Demand: The Case for Com-munity Medical Resiliency." The George Washington University, Home-land Security Policy Institute, Belfer Center for Science and International Affairs, Harvard University.

http://belfercenter.ksg.harvard.edu/publication/20358/supply_and_demand.html?breadcrumb=%2Fexperts%2F39%2Farnold_bogis (accessed July 25, 2011).

Mann, James. 2004. "THE ARMAGEDDON PLAN—During the Reagan Era Dick Cheney and Donald Rumsfeld were Key Players in a Clandestine Program Designed to Install a New 'President' in the Event of a Nuclear Attack." *The Atlantic Monthly*: 71.

National Commission on Terrorist Attacks upon the United States. 2004. *The 9/11 Commission Report: Final Report of the National Commission on Terror-ist Attacks Upon the United States*. New York: Norton.

New York City Department of Health and Mental Hygiene. "Healthcare Emergency Preparedness Program (HEPP): NYC Healthcare PREPARES." http://www.nyc.gov/html/doh/html/bhpp/bhpp.shtml (accessed July 25, 2011).

New York City Office of Emergency Management. 2005. "One Year Later…" http://www.nyc.gov/html/oem/downloads/pdf/annual_report_pg18revised.pdf (accessed July 25, 2011).

New York City Office of Emergency Management. 2007. "Biennial Report 2007." http://www.nyc.gov/html/oem/downloads/pdf/biennial_report_final_web.pdf (accessed July 25, 2011).

The Times of India. 2008. "Ahmedabad Blast Sites Chosen with Political Icons in Mind?" *The Times of India*. http://articles.timesofindia.indiatimes.com/2008-07-27/india/27902892_1_three-blasts-maninagar-city-areas (accessed July 25, 2011).

U.S. General Accounting Office. 1999. "Combating Terrorism Analysis of Federal Counterterrorist Exercises: Briefing Report to Congressional Re-questers." http://www.gao.gov/archive/1999/ns99157b.pdf (accessed July 28, 2011).